Senescence!
Defined p. 8
Used in ways incompatible w/ defn.
9, 16, 23 (wld be better defn)
28, 41

A Means to an End

WORKS BY WILLIAM R. CLARK

The Experimental Foundations of Modern Immunology

At War Within: The Double-Edged Sword of Immunity

Sex and the Origins of Death

The New Healers: The Promise and Problems of Molecular Medicine in the Twenty-First Century

A Means to an End

The Biological Basis of
Aging and Death

William R. Clark

New York   Oxford
OXFORD UNIVERSITY PRESS
1999

Oxford University Press

Oxford   New York
Athens   Auckland   Bangkok   Bogotá   Buenos Aires
Calcutta   Cape Town   Chennai   Dar es Salaam
Delhi   Florence   Hong Kong   Istanbul   Karachi
Kuala Lumpur   Madrid   Melbourne   Mexico City
Mumbai   Nairobi   Paris   São Paulo   Singapore
Taipei   Tokyo   Toronto   Warsaw

and associated companies in
Berlin   Ibadan

Copyright © 1999 by Oxford University Press

Published by Oxford University Press, Inc.
198 Madison Avenue, New York, New York 10016

Oxford is a registered trademark of Oxford University Press

Library of Congress Cataloging-in-Publication Data
Clark, William R., 1938–
A means to an end : the biological basis of aging and death /
by William R. Clark.
p.   cm.   Includes bibliographical references and index.
ISBN 0-19-512593-2
1. Cells—Aging. 2. Apoptosis. I. Title.
QH608.C53   1999
612.6'7—dc21   98–18878

3 5 7 9 8 6 4

Printed in the United States of America
on acid-free paper

For Erica
TMD

Contents

Acknowledgments

As always, a number of people have contributed to the making of this book. Kirk Jensen at Oxford University Press urged me to write on this topic in the first place, and has provided valuable guidance throughout. I have profited greatly from advice and inspiration from several colleagues: James Carey, Rita Effros, Edie Gralla, Caleb Finch, David Kirk, David Reznick, and Joan Valentine, among others.

The length of human life, according to the Greeks, was in the hands of the Fates, or Moerae. These three sisters, daughters of the Goddess of the Night, measured out the beginning, the middle, and the end of each life. Klothos spun the threads from which destinies could be woven, incorporating fibers of good or evil, happiness or tragedy into each thread. Lachesis apportioned these threads to each individual at the hour of birth, determining their length, which determined the length of each life. The third sister, Atropos—she who could not be turned aside— guarded the dread scissors that were used to cut each thread, defining the moment of death.

It is said that the three sisters were present at the birth of the great hero Meleagros, son of Oineus. Klothos spun the noblest of threads for his lifeline. Lachesis selected among these to assure his status as a hero among men. But Atropos measured her scissors along this line, and predicted he would live only as long as the log that was on the fire at his birth. At this pronouncement Meleagros' mother, Althaea, snatched the log from the flames. Years later, in a fit of anger, she threw the log back on the fire. The scissors descended, and cut the beautiful thread, so lovingly woven into a life. . . .

Introduction

The awareness that we are growing old may be uniquely human. Perhaps other animals, particularly some of the higher mammals with rudimentary cognitive function, may be aware that they are slowing down in many ways, unable to keep up with others in their group, less able to find food or capture prey, slower to move away from danger or a predator. But we doubt they understand the full implications of the process. Humans do. Only we wonder how Lachesis measures out her thread; only we want to know the nature of Atropos's scisssors. Alone among the animal species that inhabit this planet, we are endowed with consciousness, an awareness of self—where we came from, and where we are going. We alone know, only too well, that the endpoint of aging is death. This drives a concern in us about the inner workings of the aging process—senescence—that is completely lacking in other species.

For some, old age is a time of peace and joy, of reflection on life's bountifulness, a time to contemplate the only immortality we can know: the lives of our children and grandchildren. With luck and a little attention to diet and exercise, we can maintain our ability to engage both physically and mentally in those lives, and in our community of friends. But it is not so for all of us. Genetics, accident, the "luck of the draw"—all of this can play against us in our later years, depriving us of the ability to participate fully and meaningfully in the world around us. All of us have this fear as we sense old age approaching, for it can happen to anyone. And at some level, even in the lucky ones, this fear never really goes away, because we know from observing other lives that at any moment our fate could change.

So it is in a sense fear that drives us to study aging, to try to understand it; to name its parts, to unravel how they work and how it all fits together. Organized attempts to study aging in a systematic way were slow in getting started: The first professional societies dedicated to promoting basic research in senescence and aging (gerontology) and a medical specialty dealing with the problems of the aged (geriatrics) were not formed until the 1940s. As with any new field, the early years of the study of aging were filled with confusion and uncertainty. The aging process seems enormously complicated, involving complex changes in virtually every different cell type in the body. Graying hair, failing eyesight, declining physical ability and mental capacity—each of these seems like a separate physiological process, each with its own biochemical and genetic regulation.

The study of aging has some intriguing similarities to the study of cancer, and these may be instructive. For most of its clinical history, cancer was viewed as a thousand or more different diseases, at least as many different cancers as there were different cell types in the body, each requiring different treatment, each with its own outcome. But today our view of cancer is radically different. What we see now are the incredible similarities of cancer. Nearly all cancers involve mutations in a limited number of genes distributed throughout all cells in the body. This knowledge has provided a completely new basis for designing new strategies for both the detection and the treatment of cancer, strategies that are already finding their way to the clinic. The lesson from cancer that we can apply to aging is the need to understand physiological processes at their most fundamental level, at the level of the very genes that regulate it. Complex organisms like humans are composed of individual cells, and that is where the aging process begins. The aging of any organism is a reflection of the cumulative senescence of its component cells. The enormous variety of cell types in the human body, each with its own peculiar aging characteristics, or aging "phenotype," might seem to confound the search for common cellular aging mechanisms. But just as complexity in cancer came to be viewed as derangements in a limited number of genes operating in all cells, so too may senescence.

These new views of cancer and aging are part of the new field of human medicine called molecular medicine, which is in turn the fruit of basic research throughout this century in biochemistry, genetics, and molecular biology. Completion of the Human Genome Project early in the next century will eventually make it possible to identify each of the key genes involved in human aging. We will then be able to dissect senescence and aging at a level never before possible. In the past, we have had to approach aging much as the proverbial blind men approach elephants, describing it from without, in fragmented terms, trying to guess the meaning and origin of each component, with only the dimmest of views of the larger picture.

But that is about to change; soon we will see the thread of our lives—once thought to be spun, woven, and cut by fate—from a new perspective, from the inside of our own DNA. The guesswork will be gone; the view will be spectacular. What will we do with this information? How will we use it? All of us need to be engaged in a discussion of this and every other aspect of molecular medicine as we enter the next century, the next millennium. Aging is a wonderful place to start. In this book we will take a close look at what molecular medicine and its underlying sciences have to tell us about this most mysterious and fascinating of human biological processes.

A Means to an End

1

Aging, Senescence, and Lifespan

We are all aware of aging in humans from our earliest years, through normal, daily contacts with family members, neighbors, and others who have reached an advanced age. Perhaps because aging seems such an intuitively obvious phenomenon, it was quite late in becoming an object of formal study. Magical cures and restorative waters aside, the first serious scientific studies of aging did not get under way until the early part of the present century. The initial pace of research in the entire field of aging was slow; respectable scientists and physicians were doubtless deterred by the unsavory history of quack remedies and practices aimed at increasing human lifespan that had characterized the previous several centuries, as well as the first part of the twentieth century.

Perhaps we felt we didn't need a bunch of highly trained professionals telling us about getting old. We recognize it when the first signs appear in our own bodies—usually earlier than we might have expected from observing others. Elderly people look and behave differently than people in the early and peak years of their lives

(Table 1.1). They become wizened and gray, and slower to respond both physically and mentally to things around them. They appear smaller and, in fact, are: Both skeletal and muscle mass decrease, often significantly, after age fifty or so. Even the brain gets smaller, shrinking by up to 10 percent in women, and slightly more in men. All of the major organs and physiological systems undergo a gradual decline with increasing age. None of these changes is in itself a *cause* of aging; they are all the result of the aging process.

Table 1.1. *Changes Associated With Aging in Humans*

Parameter	Change
Size	Height and weight decrease in both men and women, especially after age 60, due mostly to losses of muscle and bone.
Metabolism	Gradual diminution in metabolic rate after age 30.
Skin and hair	Loss of subcutaneous fat; appearance of wrinkles, pigmentation. Graying of hair at all body sites; loss on top of head; some facial hair may increase. Nails thicken.
Heart and cardiovascular function	Some thickening of heart muscle, but no obvious diminution of pumping function in undiseased heart. Resting heart rate unchanged. Widespread cardiovascular disease after age 50; leading cause of death in both sexes.
Organ physiology	Kidney, lung, and pancreas functions diminish. Atrophy of skeletomuscular system; bone and joint problems.
Reproductive function	Female reproductive function ends at menopause; male function compromised as testosterone levels drop after age 50 or so.
Senses	Vision impairment in both sexes. Hearing, smell, and taste affected; more pronounced in men. Sense of touch only modestly affected.
Immune function	Gradual decrease in T-cell responses; increase in autoimmunity; increased susceptibility to cancer.
Neurobiology	Loss of brain cells; shrinkage of brain; physical response to stimuli slowed; learning and memory impaired; some degree of senile dementia common after age 70.

Some age-dependent changes are psychologically distressing but have little clinical impact; degeneration of the skin is a good example. Skin changes are one of the most externally visible and irrefutable signs of aging. Skin becomes thinner with age, largely because of loss of subcutaneous fat. It loses elasticity and tone because of changes in collagen, the major protein of all connective tissue, and becomes wrinkled because of both collagen changes and an increased production of a protein called elastin. Uneven distribution of the pigment melanin can result in so-called "age spots," and the skin becomes increasingly dry as sweat and oil glands gradually lose function. All of these changes associated with the normal aging process are greatly accelerated by exposure to sunlight; compare the texture of the skin on the buttocks of an elderly person with skin on the face or arms, for example. But aside from occasional skin cancers, which (with the exception of deadly malignant melanoma) are relatively harmless and easily treated, aged skin is biologically nearly as effective as young skin, and causes no threat to health or well-being.

But of course "clinical impact" does not always adequately describe the tremendous psychological impact many of the changes associated with aging can bring. Mental confusion and slowness to respond to simple questions do not at all imply an unawareness of, or indeed a painful embarrassment about, one's diminished mental capacities. Increasing weakness and a tendency to fall can be not only physically dangerous, but can drive many older individuals to become increasingly immobile through fear of embarrassing themselves. Perhaps most humiliating of all the assaults of old age is urinary incontinence. This condition, affecting some fifteen million Americans, is a major factor in the self-imposed social isolation of many elderly people. The overall loss of the ability to control the image of ourselves seen by others may be one of the most devastating changes of growing old, ranking with the fear of death itself as a psychological toll of aging.

In terms of human morbidity and mortality, age-associated degenerative changes in the cardiovascular system are probably most critical, for the obvious reason that all of the other cells of the body are dependent on a constant blood supply for food and oxygen. The death of a relatively small number of brain cells through lack of oxygen, and the consequent inability of the brain to coordinate physiological activities in the rest of the body, can occur within minutes of a serious heart attack, and result in death of the entire organism. Cardiovascular disease is the leading cause of death in people over fifty years of age in the United States and most of the industrialized world. To some extent this reflects the fact that other causes of death have been brought under control; each time one cause of death is reduced, another emerges to take its place.

The vascular changes leading to coronary artery disease can occur in arteries elsewhere in the body as well, resulting in a variety of other serious complications such as stroke or gangrene. These changes are largely due to atherosclerosis (literally, sludge-hardening), in which the inner lining of the arteries delivering blood throughout the body become thicker and less flexible, and the lumen itself becomes clogged with oxidized fatty deposits that include cholesterol. The result is reduced blood flow to all parts of the body. Interestingly, the pumping function of the heart muscle itself, in the absence of cardiovascular disease, does not weaken significantly with age.

We are also more open to attack from the outside as we get older. The immune system is less able to fight off invasion by microbial pathogens, and even begins slowly to attack the body itself in the collection of disorders known as autoimmune disease. The thymus gland, which plays a key role in the development of an important disease-fighting white blood cell called the T (for thymus-derived) cell, begins to atrophy at about the time of sexual maturity; the loss of this immunological "master organ" doubtless impairs T-cell function in the body over time. In addition to playing a direct role in defense against infectious disease, T cells also play a role in regulating many other components of the immune system. Thus the well-documented diminution of T-cell function with age may be a major cause of decreased immune defense against disease. The increased incidence of autoimmune disease with age could be related to the gradual loss of T-cell regulatory function, or it may be due to production of "self" molecules altered with age that the immune system comes to regard as foreign.

Reproductive capacity in most species changes markedly with age. It is largely controlled by hormones produced in the pituitary gland of the brain, and the pattern of synthesis and release of these hormones changes in an age-dependent manner. In virtually every species, the degenerative changes associated with aging are substantially held back until reproductive maturity. In mammals generally, the changes in reproductive capacity with age are more pronounced in females than in males. The sudden changes brought on in human females at menopause are a striking example of the close link between reproduction and senescence. But human males also experience a decrease in reproductive ability with age. The necessity to defer age-related physical decline in all systems until reproductive maturity is a key to understanding the basic biology of aging.

Not only is the aging process complex in terms of the spectrum of changes that occur across multiple organs and tissues, but it also seems to begin at different times in different people, and to proceed at differing paces. We all know of people who look old "before their time," or others who look ten or even twenty years younger than they actually are. Some people turn gray in their thirties, while others die at eighty with a full head of deeply colored hair. Wrinkles set in at different times in different people. Some people in their nineties seem to have lost very little of their hair or their mental capacities (not that the two traits are connected), while others in their fifties cannot recall a friend's name, or remember why they walked into a room. Does this reflect a difference in the aging program itself, or a difference in the interaction of natural aging mechanisms with variable environmental factors? This is one of the most fundamental questions addressed by those who study aging.

While the changes associated with aging are quite obvious in humans, it is rare to observe the aging process at work in animal populations living in the wild, because of the very high level, in most species (including pre-modern humans), of accidental death. Accidental death will be an important concept in our considerations of the aging and longevity of individual organisms. We will explore accidental death below in some detail in terms of its associated cellular events, but here let us define it at the organismal level simply as death from causes lying outside the individual organism—things like being eaten by a predator, starvation or infectious disease, as well as fatal physical accidents. It is to be distinguished from what we might call, for lack of a better term, natural death—death that results from purely internal causes such as genetic disease, heart attack, cancer, or other age-related disorders.

When talking about the basic biology of aging, as opposed to its outward physical and behavioral manifestations, it is common to talk about something called senescence. Senescence is here defined as the increasing likelihood of death of an individual with advancing age. On one level, such a statement may seem so intuitively obvious that it scarcely bears writing down, let alone dedicating an entire book to its explanation. Yet as we will see, senescence is in fact one of the least understood processes in all of biology, and thus one of the least understood aspects of human medicine. The simplest statements about it often provoke seemingly endless debate and discussion among those who study it.

What precisely is meant by "an increasing likelihood of death with advancing age?" What we mean is that for any defined increment of time—a calendar year of life in the case of humans, for example—the probability of death in the $n+1$ time increment is demonstrably greater then the probability of death in the nth increment; the probability of death in the $n+2$ increment is greater than the probability in the $n+1$ increment; and so on. But notice that this definition of senescence does not mention any of the characteristics that we associate with aging per se; it mentions only death. This has important implications for understanding the evolution of senescence. One of the things we will try to establish about the various forms of natural death—death from senescence—is that ultimately all of them involve information embedded in and controlled through our DNA. Senescence can be explained and understood at the cellular and molecular level, as well as appreciated in the context of the whole organism.

Most humans in industrialized societies die either directly or indirectly from the causes of senescence, as do some wild animals kept in zoos or laboratories where they are largely protected from accidental death. From a purely biological point of view, senescence is nature's backup plan; if we do not die from external accidental causes, then ultimately we will die from the cumulative effects of internal senescence. But accidental and natural death are intimately intertwined in the life history of every species; individuals die from one cause or the other, but very often senescence—in the form of cancer or cardiovascular disease or a genetic disorder—increases an organism's susceptibility to disease and accidental death. The gradual physical weakening that accompanies aging will make an animal more likely to be caught by a predator; diminished immune capacity can make us more susceptible to infectious disease. Moreover, different forms of senescence can interact; decreased immune function, for example, can also make us more susceptible to purely internal diseases such as cancer. It is complications like these that are best sorted out by beginning our study of aging and death not at the cellular or molecular level, but at the very opposite end of the biological spectrum—in large populations.

Death in a crowd: Senescence and lifespan in populations

At a population level, aging and death are often analyzed in terms of survival curves, examples of which are shown in Figure 1.1. In these curves, we are looking at the survival over time of some large initial number—a cohort—of newborn members of the same species. Such curves display death from both accident and senescence inextricably mingled together; in populations living in the wild it is rarely possible to separate them. Curve A in this figure is thus entirely theoretical, and would never obtain in the real world. It is what we would imagine a survival curve to look like if senescence were the only cause of death in a population. There would be little or no death from senescence until that point in their overall lifespan where individuals in the cohort normally produce at least a replacement number of offspring, that is, the number of offspring needed to provide enough reproduc-

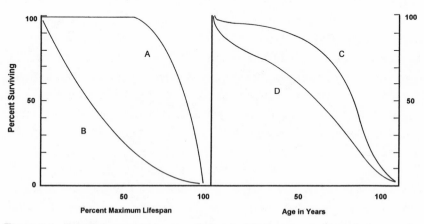

Figure 1.1. Population survival curves: theoretical (*left*) and actual (*right*). See text for explanation of curves *A–D*.

tively competent adult individuals to maintain or expand the species in its natural habitat. That point in life (set here arbitrarily at about 70 percent of lifespan), and the number of requisite offspring, is different in different species, and can even change within a species as conditions in the environment change. But already we have incorporated an important theoretical point into our hypothetical curve: Significant senescence does not set in until reproductive maturity has been achieved, or if it does, it must be offset by processes that effectively neutralize it.

Once individuals have reached sexual maturity, and have had an adequate opportunity to reproduce, senescence would begin to operate, and individuals would start to die, either directly or indirectly, from senescence. These deaths would occur more or less randomly, across some fairly brief period of time. Survival curves of this type approximate a rectangle, the deviation of the descending leg from the vertical indicating the efficiency of the senescence process; human females may live fifty or more years beyond menopause, whereas a female salmon may live only a day or two after spawning. We assume that in a natural population, death from accidental causes will continue and perhaps even accelerate during this portion of the curve as well. And it is in the descending portion of the curve that the definition presented earlier about senescence is in full operation; for an individual managing to survive to any point on this descent, the likelihood of death will be greater at subsequent time points than it was at preceding time points.

Curve B in the figure is also entirely theoretical, and typifies a population in which death from senescence does not occur at all. Death of the entire cohort in this case results from accidental causes, such as starvation, predation, or physical trauma, and is essentially exponential; if it were plotted logarithmically, instead of arithmetically as shown here, the survival curve would be a straight line as long as environmental conditions remain constant. What this means is that across *any* fixed interval of time, beginning at the moment of birth, a constant proportion of the surviving members of the selected cohort will die. The shape of this curve of course could be altered somewhat if, for example, older members of the species have a reduced susceptibility to accidental death because of increased size or some age-dependent physiological change. The survival curves for some invertebrate organisms, particularly certain insects and aquatic species like *Hydra* and most sea anemones, actually approach curve B rather closely.

Interestingly, curve B looks very much like a survival curve for inanimate objects that wear out from mechanical usage. In a study described in Alex Comfort's book, *The Biology of Senescence*, a virtually identical curve was generated by following the "survival" of a large cohort of glass tumblers in a public cafeteria. A fairly constant proportion of glasses disappeared each week from accidents—dropping by customers or employees, and breakage in the cleaning or drying process. Similar "exponential decay" curves would be generated by following the fate of any number of other objects subjected to random destruction through accident.

Curve C is a reasonable facsimile of the expected survival of human beings born in the United States in the last decades of the twentieth century; like most survival curves, it displays death caused by a mixture of accident and senescence. We can expect in the twenty-first century that many people will continue to die by accidental means—infectious disease, physical accidents, and the like—but that the majority will die of senescence, and because of increased susceptibility to accidental death caused by senescence. Note that this curve is much closer in shape to curve A than curve B; it is more "rectangularized." That is because senescence is a major factor in human mortality today. Were we to plot survival curves for certain other large mammals, such as whales or elephants, they would approximate that of humans more than they would the survival curves for invertebrates, or even small mammals such as field mice or voles, which also look more like curve B. Curve C is also similar to the survival exhibited by many animals maintained in zoos, or even invertebrates reared in the laboratory. By protecting these organisms from predators and providing them with food and an opportunity to exercise, their survival curves can be radically shifted from a curve A-like to a curve B-like form. Finally, curve C is similar to curves plotting the survival of complex mechanical devices such as automobiles, where there would be a limited amount of loss from accident at all stages in the "life history" of a cohort of cars, compounded by losses from a variety of internal mechanical failures beginning at some point, leading to a sharp decline in the survival rate.

The point of initiation of senescence in curve C is not obvious; we are plotting only the disappearance of individuals with age, from the cumulative effects of accident and senescence; we have arbitrarily set the point at which senescence becomes a major factor in mortality at about 60 percent of total lifespan, which is probably not far off for humans. We do not know exactly when significant senescence per se sets in in humans; tests of athletic ability in males suggest physical performance begins to decline noticeably somewhere in the late twenties. Senescence resulting in significant mortality is delayed in all species until at least the beginning of the reproductive period. Given that humans are sexually mature in their early teens, and ten years is probably a reasonable reproductive period, we might expect to see senescence setting in at around the mid- to late twenties. On the other hand, it was pointed out early in this century that the growth rate of human cells in vitro ("in glass"; i.e., outside the human body) slows down substantially almost immediately after birth, which might indicate the onset of some sort of senescent program. Because we do not have an unambiguous test or "marker" for senescence, particularly in humans, we cannot at present detect its onset. Its conclusion, on the other hand, is quite clear.

Note also that the survival curve for humans tends to flatten out somewhat at the very end. This feature is real, and not due to careless curve drawing. Detailed analysis of human survival in many countries around the world has shown that the likelihood of death across a given time interval decreases somewhat with very advanced age—those who survive longer survive the longest! The same thing is seen in animal populations. One of the most impressive studies was that reported by James Carey and his associates on Mediterranean fruit flies in 1992. Carey studied the mortality pattern in over one million flies, lending his work a statistical accuracy rarely achieved in biological studies. He found that the mortality rate (the percentage of survivors in a cohort dying at any given time) decreased markedly among the last 0.1 percent of surviving flies. This phenomenon represents an important exception to the definition of senescence set out earlier, as the increased likelihood of death with age; for the last few survivors of any given cohort, the likelihood of death actually decreases with time. It does not, however, go to zero.

In both flies and humans, the most likely explanation of the "tailing off" effect in populations is genetic heterogeneity within the species. It should be noted that in both cases, the data tell us what is happening at the population level, not at the individual level; it is entirely possible—indeed, likely—that for any given individual, the likelihood of death in fact continues to increase in a more or less steady fashion throughout latter stages of life. As we will discuss throughout the rest of this book, senescence is at least in part under genetic control. There are many reasons for believing this, but one of the simplest is that genetically identical twins die much closer in time to one another than do fraternal twins or non-twin siblings. The slowing of mortality with advanced age might reflect the fact that those alive toward the very end of the human survival curve—the "oldest old"*— represent individuals in whom the senescence process has been operating more slowly all along, or who are genetically less susceptible to some of the major senescence factors in humans. We know, for example, that heart failure and cancer as causes of death are up to ten times less frequent in the oldest old; those genetically more susceptible to these diseases presumably succumbed to them during the "normal old" period of sixty-five to eigty-five years of age.

Curve D is a facsimile of a survival curve for humans born in the last decade of the nineteenth century. What is particularly evident here is the substantially higher rate of infant and childhood mortality, largely caused by infectious diseases, and a somewhat greater rate of loss of individuals in their reproductive years, from a wide range of health problems and workplace accidents. Overall, the curve is much less "rectangular" than curve C. But note that although the average lifespan is quite different from that in curve C, the age of the oldest individuals dying in the cohorts born in the last years of the nineteenth and twentieth centuries is not terribly different, and in fact may not be different at all. That is because in both populations, the individuals dying in the final decade of life are dying largely from senescence, which seems to have a common endpoint for all members of the species.

This brings up a concept alluded to in our discussion so far, but not fully explained: <u>maximum possible lifespan</u>. Although important to

---

*Because old age is not a single, easily definable stage of life, demographers have found it useful to divide old age into several distinct phases. Throughout this book, we will use the following nomenclature to define stages in the aging of humans. Youngest-old: 50–65 years; old: 65–85 years; oldest-old: 85–99 years; centenarians: 100 years and older.

both basic scientists and demographers, maximum lifespan is a bit of a slippery concept. It could be defined as the last documentable point on the survival curve for a species at which an individual has been observed to be alive. It is often defined as the average age of some small proportion—1 percent or so—of the longest living members of a species. We do not know exactly where along the age axis in curves C and D the true maximum lifespan lies for humans; it is certainly closer to the "three-score and ten" of the 90th Psalm than to the 900-plus years attributed to some of the Old Testament patriarchs. Most demographers would probably agree it lies somewhere between 110 and 120 years (Table 1.2).

Maximum lifespan varies enormously among the species inhabiting the earth today, from a matter of days to hundreds of years. For a few very large mammals, including humans, maximum lifespan can be estimated by observing populations in their natural habitat. Anecdotes and "common wisdom" about human lifespan confused the issue until late in the last century. Although the great French naturalist Georges Buffon had recognized in the mid-eighteenth century that human beings, regardless of their race or social station, only rarely lived beyond a hundred years, accounts of lifespans of as many as 165 years continued to be believed by eminent authorities well into the twentieth century.

However, a classical and detailed study published in 1873 by the amateur British demographer William Thoms debunked almost every such claim, and, based on his analysis of insurance company records and various birth and death registries, Thoms correctly concluded that Buffon's upper limit of 100 years was substantially accurate. More recent tales of extremely long-lived individuals, for example in the Caucasus region of Georgia and neighboring countries, continue to surface to this day, but do not stand up to close scrutiny. (Josef Stalin was from this region, and apparently enthusiastically promoted claims of unusual longevity by his compatriots.) Demographers examine all such claims meticulously, and find that very old people are often confused about their age. Unimpeachable documentation is required before recognizing the longevity claims of anyone over 100 years old.

For mammalian species other than humans, as mentioned earlier, maximum lifespan is normally observed only in animals kept in zoos or maintained in laboratories, where accidental death can be controlled. But the rather startling fact is that it is still there in these lat-

Table 1.2. *Maximum Possible Lifespans for Selected Species*

Common Name	Maximum Lifespan (Years)
Marine bivalve	220
(Giant) tortoise	180
Human	122
Elephant	70
Halibut	60
Orangutan	58
Chimpanzee	55
(Bateleur) eagle	55
Hippopotamus	54
Horse	45
Gorilla	40
Baboon	36
Polar bear	34
Cat	30
Cow	30
Fruit bat	30
Tiger	26
Dog	20
Squirrel monkey	20
Sparrow	13
Tree shrew	8
Rat	3.9
Mouse	3.5
Mole	1.9
European shrew	0.3

ter cases, and it is remarkably constant within a species even though only rarely, if ever, reached in the wild. On the other hand, maximum lifespan can be quite different between physically similar species living in the same ecological niche, and these differences are stably transmitted from one generation to the next. This constancy and heritability of maximum lifespan within a species, and its independence of environmental factors—first recognized by Buffon in the eighteenth century—can be taken as a priori evidence that maximum lifespan is at least in part a genetically determined trait.

Trying to understand the factors that determine maximum possible lifespan is one of the most puzzling aspects of the overall study of senescence and death. For some single-cell organisms such as yeast, it is not even definable in calendar time, but rather in a total number of cell divisions. That is, at "birth" the cell has a preset average number of divisions that it can undergo before succumbing to the ravages of senescence. The length of time required to complete these divisions may vary considerably; it may be slowed down or speeded up at the extremes of temperature tolerated by the cell. The lifespan of many invertebrate species is also markedly affected by temperature. Moreover, some single-cell organisms are able to form cysts, spore-like structures that are metabolically inert, when conditions in the environment are insufficient to support life, such as ambient temperatures outside the tolerated range, insufficient food or water, or too much or too little salt. Cells can stay in this death-like state for months or years, and when restored to an active form continue the completion of their predetermined number of cell divisions as if nothing had happened. If a cohort were split in half, and half allowed to encyst, the encysted half, when "revived," could still be alive years after all cells in the other half of the cohort had died. This definition of cellular lifespan based on a number of replications rather than calendar time is found in many cells throughout the animal kingdom, including many human cells removed from the body and grown in incubators.

The variation in maximum lifespan in multicellular animals is, to a first approximation, a function of how long after birth senescence must be delayed in order to permit at least a replacement level of reproductive activity (including protection and rearing of offspring, in those species where this occurs.) As is evident in Figure 1.1, a clear distinction exists between maximum lifespan and average lifespan. The average lifespan in a defined cohort is the age at which 50 percent of the cohort is still alive. Depending on the population under consideration, average lifespan may be determined almost exclusively by accidental cell death or by some combination of accidental death and programmed death (senescence). Maximum lifespan, on the other hand— and this is a very important distinction—is determined *solely by the rate and timing of the onset of senescence, and not by accidental death.*

How does this make sense, given the defn on p. 8.

16

Numerous attempts have been made to correlate maximum lifespan with other attributes of multicellular animals, in order to gain insight into the genetic basis of maximum lifespan. There is a rough correlation of maximum lifespan with body weight (Fig. 1.2), but there are obvious exceptions (compare cows and elephants with humans and rhesus monkeys, for example, or bats and sparrows with mice). August Weismann, the great German biologist and one of the founders of reproductive genetics, pointed out at the end of the nineteenth century that queen ants and the males who breed with them are similar in size, but the former has a maximum lifespan of several years, whereas the males live only a few weeks. The same is true of bees, medflies, and other insects. Birds and small rodents are similar in size, but the former often have maximum lifespans of a dozen years, whereas rats, mice, and voles rarely have maximum lifespan values in excess of three to four years. Weismann correctly inferred that senescence is probably regulated by some internal program that is typical of each species, unrelated in any direct way to the environment, and that greater size

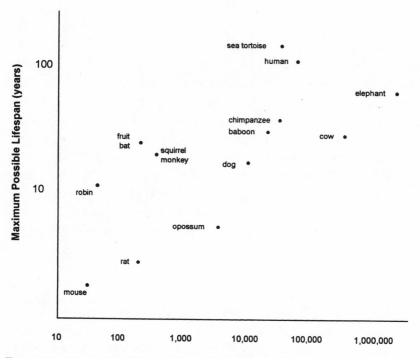

Figure 1.2. Correlation of body weight with maximum lifespan.

results from, rather than causes, delayed senescence.* Correlations of size with maximal lifespan improve somewhat when brain size in relation to body weight is factored in, but still leave a great deal to be desired. Moreover, no one has come up with a reasonable proposal of how the size of an organism and/or its brain could affect longevity.

A second intriguing correlation of maximum lifespan has been found with metabolic rate, the rate at which an organism must burn food and oxygen to produce the energy needed to operate its cells. This parameter, too, correlates roughly with size, in that smaller animals must consume much more food per unit time and per unit body weight than larger animals. This means that they also must deal with a higher level of metabolic waste products per unit time and body weight. As we will see in a later chapter, some of these by-products—especially of oxygen—are toxic, and are a major contributing factor in cellular senescence.

Although relatively constant for a species living in its natural environment, for many single-cell and even multicellular organisms, maximum lifespan can be shortened or lengthened in the laboratory by manipulations as simple as changing the growth temperature. This is presumably due to alterations in metabolic rates, reinforcing the notion that maximum lifespan is governed at least in part by metabolic processes. Maximum lifespan can also be altered by dietary manipulation, mainly by restricting the intake of calories. Studies of this type began shortly after the turn of the present century. Limiting food intake in a wide range of laboratory organisms—from single-cell organisms through rats and mice—was found to increase maximal lifespan, in some cases up to double the normal maximum lifespan. In warm-blooded animals, it is the only known way to modulate maximum lifespan. The dietary restriction effect was most pronounced if restriction was initiated prior to the reproductive period, although restriction of caloric intake in older animals can also be effective in prolonging lifespan. Extreme restriction, of course, may actually hasten

---

*Obviously, for many social insects such as ants, where different members of the same species have vastly different lifespans, genetic programs controlling senescence must be under different controls or have different pathways for members of the species with different social roles. But the constancy of the lifespan for these differing members still argues strongly for a genetic basis of the varying lifespans.

physical decline. Dietary restriction in young animals is almost always accompanied by growth retardation, which is largely restored if normal feeding is resumed. This fact in itself was of great interest when these experiments were first carried out, because they seemed to suggest that achievement of full body size might in some way be linked to onset of senescence. However, as with other correlations of size and longevity, this does not hold up. We will examine the relation of caloric intake to maximum lifespan in detail in Chapter 8.

Finally, there is the intriguing difference in lifespan between men and women. Currently, men in the United States and most industrialized countries have an average lifespan that is about seven years less than that for women. In Russia, the gap is slightly over ten years. This was not always so in the United States, and it is not true today in some developing countries. Prior to the middle of the last century in this country, men lived longer than women, probably due to a combination of the hazards of childbirth and the greater vulnerability of women to physical harm such as accidents and wartime deprivation. The rate of death among women in the United States giving birth today is less than 10 percent of what it was at the end of the nineteenth century. These factors still compromise the survival of women in some parts of the world.

The reason for the longer average lifespan of women in a more protected environment is unclear; it may be as simple as the fact that women, at least in the past, have smoked less, consumed less alcohol, and are in general more averse to physical risk. It is now well established that during the child-bearing years women are protected by hormones from cardiovascular disease, and they appear to have stronger immune systems; these protections are lost at menopause. But it is also possible that women have a slightly longer inherent maximum lifespan. Three of every four centenarians are women. And even at these very oldest ages, women still have a slightly greater life expectancy than do men who somehow manage to live that long. The basis for this effect is entirely unknown, but it is assumed to be related to the more important role of the female in the reproductive process. Intriguingly, a possible survival advantage to human females is seen even before birth. Significantly more fertilization events result in the creation of male embryos than female, but at birth the two sexes are just about even, with 51 percent being male, and 49 percent female.

The changes wrought in average lifespan through improvements in public health, medicine, and accident prevention are readily understandable, and certainly greatly appreciated. But maximum possible lifespan is a mystery that continues to fascinate us. The causes of human death have changed dramatically during our history as a species, but maximum lifespan, as far as we can tell, has not. As the twentieth century draws to a close, cardiovascular disease and stroke, cancer and pneumonia account for three-quarters of all human deaths. What will happen when these diseases are overcome? Our previous biological history would suggest that maximum lifespan will not change much. But can we be absolutely certain this is true? And what then would we die of? Is there an ultimate cause of human death responsible for the apparent fixity of human maximum lifespan? Or would all human death be accidental? We will explore these questions in the following chapters.

2

The Nature of Cellular Senescence and Death

For the most part in this book, we will be examining both senescence and death at the level of individual cells, and for a very good reason. Cells are the biological equivalent of the atoms of chemistry, in the sense that they are the smallest thing of which we can say, "This is alive." It follows, then, that cells are also the smallest thing of which we can say, "This is not alive; this is dead." Senescence and death in an organism—whether the organism under consideration is itself a single cell, like a yeast or a bacterium, or a complex multicellular organism like a human being—is ultimately a reflection of the senescence and death of individual cells. The outward manifestations of aging are enormously complex, and this has led in the past almost to a feeling of helplessness in studying the underlying processes. Formerly, many of those who studied aging felt that each component of aging—wrinkled skin, cataracts, gray hair, or diminished mental function—must reflect a different underlying mechanism. Yet if we understand that all of the cells in a complex organism like a human being are for the most part similar, with only a small portion of their endowment dedicated to making them different, we might gain hope that in fact a reasonably limited number of fundamental processes are at work in the senescence and death of individual cells. The way in which these processes manifest themselves may be determined by only a tiny fraction of a cell's genetic endowment.

What do senescence and death mean at the level of a single cell? Even under the most sophisticated microscope, there is very little difference in the outward appearance of a cell at the moment of its death and one that is perfectly healthy, just as there is little difference in superficial appearance between someone who has just died and someone who has just fallen asleep. So how do we know when a cell is dead? This is an important question, because the death of a living organism begins with the death of a portion of its cells. What exactly is it that is missing in a cell when it dies? What qualities define a cell as being alive, the absence of which would make it dead? What makes a cell old?

There are many criteria used to define life in a cell. Perhaps the most important is the ability to consume energy-rich materials (nutrients), extract the energy from them, and then use that energy to carry out the various chemical reactions supporting life within the cell. All living things do this; it is the process known as metabolism. Cells use energy derived in this fashion—metabolic energy—to form their structural and functional components, to reproduce themselves, and to respond to the environment, for example, to move about in search of food or to escape from predators or poisons. All single-cell organisms, and multicellular organisms that do not generate their own heat, are also dependent on the direct absorption of thermal energy from the sun. The biochemical reactions necessary to extract energy from food simply do not work well as temperatures drop toward the freezing point of water, because these reactions are always dependent for their chemical integrity on water in the liquid rather than the solid state. Warm-blooded animals use metabolic energy together with ambient solar energy to keep their internal temperatures within a reasonable working range.

For most biologists, then, the various definitions of life can nearly all be traced back to the presence within individual cells of an active metabolism—an ability to extract energy from the environment and use it to carry out the range of biological functions that we call life. Cellular death can then largely be defined in terms of the absence— but it must be the complete absence—of an active metabolism. Senescence is the sequence of events connecting these two states through time in the life history of an individual: the conversion of a metabolically active cell, through a series of genetically controlled events, to a cell no longer capable of metabolic function.

To understand how, or at least why, senescence and death came into being, it will be useful first to try to understand the various roles the death of cells plays in nature, and also the manner in which cells die. There are, as it turns out, two quite different ways in which cells die. The first form of death is what is usually referred to as accidental cell death. As with whole organisms, accidental death in cells occurs entirely in response to conditions outside the cell: insufficient food or water, too much or too little heat, chemical poisoning, physical trauma, or simply being eaten by a predator. For the vast majority of biologically simpler organisms, many of which are themselves only single cells, accidental cell death is the predominant form of cellular death. In fact, for the evolutionarily most primitive single-cell organisms, the prokaryotes (cells that do not have a nucleus, represented on the earth today by the bacteria), accidental cell death is the *only* form of death. Prokaryotes were the first cells to appear on earth—the very first form of life—and reigned for about a billion years before other life forms evolved from them. They remain today one of the largest components of the earth's biomass. An important feature of prokaryotes then and now is that each cell has only a single copy of a single chromosome (the string of DNA containing the genes), a condition referred to as haploid. All subsequent forms of life would have two copies each, usually of multiple different chromosomes, and are referred to as diploid. This distinction may have important implications for the genetic basis of senescence, as we shall see.

Bacteria are, from a biological point of view, potentially immortal. Each cell divides into two daughter cells in an asexual process called fission (we will examine sexual reproduction shortly.) The haploid DNA copy in a dividing (mother) cell is first doubled, and then there is a random and equal distribution of all cellular components, including the two DNA copies, into the daughters, which themselves each divide into two more cells, and so on, potentially ad infinitum. It has long been recognized that this succession of generations is not accompanied by death in any biological meaning of the word; if so, as August Weismann first pointed out in 1882, where is the corpse? True, the individual identity of the cell entering the fission event is in a sense lost, although it could be said to be present in the daughter cells, which are perfect clones of the mother. Nevertheless, there is nothing we could define biologically as cellular death associated with fission. Bacteria do not divide endlessly, of course; their rapid growth rate will quickly lead them to outstrip the ability of the environment to support them with enough food, and they will starve to death—a form of accidental cell death.

The second form of cellular death is called programmed cell death, which is the death that is required of cells as a condition of life, and the death that is the endpoint of senescence. Programmed death as we will describe it in this and subsequent chapters does not exist in prokaryotes, but it is characteristic of all of the higher life forms evolving from them. The earliest of these higher life forms (all of which are called eukaryotes, because they store their diploid chromosome sets in a true nucleus within the cell) were themselves single cells, but some of these gradually evolved into multicellular organisms which gave rise to all higher plant and animal life forms. Eukaryotic cells can die either by accidental death or by programmed death. In fact, for many eukaryotic life forms, accidental death is so likely an outcome of life that programmed death is difficult to see except in the laboratory. Among the simpler multicellular eukaryotes, accidental death is so common that some of them may produce tens of thousands of offspring at each mating, simply to assure that one or two survive to reproduce. As discussed in Chapter 3, this presents a major difficulty in understanding how senescence and programmed death could have evolved; the vast majority of offspring perish long before a senescence program could possibly come into play. Nevertheless, some small number of offspring *do* survive to adulthood in each generation, and it is these individuals we should focus on in thinking about the evolution of senescence, since they are the ones that breed.

There are a number of key differences between accidental cell death and programmed cell death. Accidental cell death can occur virtually instantly, for example, in the case of physical trauma; a cell smashed by a hammer does not go through a particularly elaborate process of dying. But other forms of accidental cell death do involve something like a process, and the process is called necrosis. The main feature of necrosis as a way of dying is that it is resisted with everything the cell under challenge has at its command. Cells that are deprived of oxygen, for example, can switch their internal metabolic pathways to those not requiring oxygen, and those deprived of nutrients may begin to burn internal stores of food until external sources become available again. Some cells may even transform themselves into a metabolically inert state that requires neither food nor oxygen; prokaryotic spores or eukaryotic cysts can remain in suspended states for months or even years.

Programmed cell death is very different. First, the "program" is not one of resistance to death, but one of active participation in the process. The death program in an individual cell may be initiated in response to external factors—signals coming from other cells in the body, for example—but the cell so instructed does not resist this signal. In one of the most common forms of programmed cell death, the cell simply sets in motion the internal cellular mechanisms necessary to complete the program in a process often referred to as cellular "suicide," or more properly, apoptosis. It is important to maintain a distinction between apoptosis and programmed cell death. The latter is defined simply as any genetically regulated program leading to the death of a cell. Apoptosis is one common way of achieving programmed cell death, but it may not be the only means.

One of the most common examples of programmed cell death in higher organisms occurs during mammalian (including human) fetal development. At about five weeks of human fetal life, what will shortly be a hand looks a good deal like a Ping-Pong paddle (Fig. 2.1 A, B). Although the future fingers can just be perceived as cartilaginous condensations along the axis of the hand, they are still connected together by a thin film of cellular webbing. Over the next week or so, the cells making up this webbing will die, very peacefully, via apoptosis. The same type of cellular suicide is seen in the development of the fetal nervous system. At a certain point, the brain and spinal cord send out enormous numbers of perfectly good nerve fibers. Some of these fibers will find organs and tissues to innervate, providing a lifelong connection between the central nervous system and the peripheral tissues. However, as many as half of the nerve fibers thus generated and flung

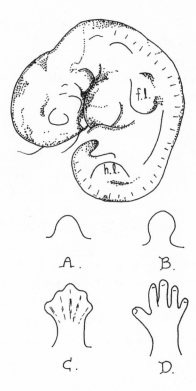

Figure 2.1. Development of the human hand. By the fifth week, the forelimb (f.l.) and hindlimb (h.l.) are apparent. Stages in forelimb development are shown below: (*A*) 5 weeks; (*B*) 5.5 weeks; (*C*) 6.5 weeks; (*D*) two months. (Drawn by Celine Park)

out to the periphery fail to establish a meaningful connection. These fibers soon die by apoptosis. This kind of programmed cell death is very common throughout the lifespan of many higher organisms.

These two ways of dying are quite distinct at the microscopic and biochemical levels as well. Eukaryotic cells are highly organized internally, with tiny intracellular organs (called organelles) that carry out all of the cells' specialized functions such as energy production and protein synthesis. These organelles are not randomly scattered throughout the cell, but have specific spatial arrangements necessary for their proper function. In cellular necrosis, the cause of death is usually insufficient cellular energy to maintain the membrane pumps that keep certain ions inside the cell, and water out. When these pumps fail, water rushes into the cell, disrupting organelles, scrambling the intracellular architecture, and finally causing the cell to burst open, rupturing its membrane. The contents of the cell spill out, and in many higher animals trigger an inflammatory response that in itself can be damaging to surrounding tissues.

In apoptosis, the intracellular architecture is not disturbed, and the cell does not rupture; rather, it fragments into small "apoptotic bodies" that, in multicellular animals, are ingested by neighboring cells. Until the moment of ingestion, organellar function inside these apoptotic bodies seems to go on more or less normally. But perhaps the most interesting feature of apoptosis occurs inside the cell's nucleus. Once a signal to commit suicide has been delivered, the DNA in the nucleus fragments into millions of tiny pieces that can no longer function to direct the activities of the cell. Although the cell may continue on for many hours after DNA fragmentation has occurred, the cell at that moment is irreversibly destined to die.

Unravelling how this death program works in cells induced to undergo apoptosis is one of the most active areas of current research in cell biology. The signal to commit suicide can also come from within the cell itself, for example, if cellular machinery set up for that purpose detects excessive DNA damage within the cell's nucleus, or determines that the cell has been invaded by a virus or has become cancerous. The intracellular events that follow receipt of an appropriate "death signal," whatever its origin, are extraordinarily complex and not yet fully understood. Sometimes the response is to commit suicide; sometimes the response (particularly for cells that are rapidly dividing) may simply be to shunt into a state of advanced senescence where they may remain for a long time. We do not yet understand how the choice between these two fates is made, or how or when the newly senescent cells will die. What is clear, however, is that this program is under very tight genetic control. Many of the genes responsible for apoptosis have been identified, and even cloned and sequenced. Given the pace of research in this field, in a few years we will likely have this program, and its regulation, dissected in considerable detail. Exactly how it fits into the overall aging process should then become quite clear.

Evolutionary Origins of Cellular Senescence

Senescence can be detected in many of the earliest eukaryotic life forms, including those which, like their prokaryotic ancestors, were (and are) single cells. Although in some ways primitive, these single-cell organisms have been very successful, and today occupy an entire evolutionary kingdom—the Protista—which includes among other things slime molds, amoebas, algae, and numerous single-cell parasites like the one that causes malaria. It seems quite likely that senescence, accompanied by obligatory death, appeared in evolution very close to the time that eukaryotes first emerged from prokaryotes. None of the protists in existence today expresses senescence exactly as we find it in more advanced multicellular animals, but there can be no question that aging was a normal part of the protist life cycle.

One trend in the evolution of early eukaryotes was simply to get larger; the freshwater ciliated protozoan called *Paramecium* is an excellent example of this trend. We imagine that a major driving force behind getting larger was the advantage it provided for becoming a predator, or perhaps fending off other would-be predators. Becoming larger also provided increased room for the development of a more sophisticated intracellular architecture, and for storage of food supplies that could be used to provide energy when extracellular food sources were scarce. But increased size brought with it a number of problems, not the least of which was supplying enough proteins to operate a cell that had become almost a million times larger in volume than the average bacterium. Proteins are made in response to instructions from the genes embedded in DNA, and there is a limit to how fast these instructions can be read and translated into the corresponding proteins. Although eukaryotes had doubled the amount of their DNA in becoming diploid, at some point in the evolution of size even this amount of DNA became inadequate to supply enough copies of the individual proteins needed to operate the cell.

What paramecia did to meet this challenge was to expand (by replication) certain portions of their total DNA allotment (their genome), and to segregate this additional DNA into a separate nucleus within the cell called the macronucleus. The randomly amplified portions of DNA stored in the macronucleus were used on a daily basis to produce all of the proteins needed to operate the cell. The micronucleus continued to house a single, pristine, diploid set of DNA-containing chromosomes within the cell that was used only in connection with sexual reproduction, as we shall see in a moment. This is the first point in evolution where we see a segregation of DNA into two biologically distinct compartments within the same organism: operational DNA and reproductive DNA. This segregation would have major implications for the life cycle of paramecia and all subsequent eukaryotes, for it would lead almost immediately to a requirement for senescence and death.

A form of senescence called replicative senescence in organisms like paramecia had been noted by cell biologists at the end of the nineteenth century, although its relation to aging in higher organisms was not recognized until the 1960s. If the evolutionarily older bacteria are placed in a large vat of growth medium, they will divide at a fixed rate essentially without limit. As long as fresh medium is added periodically, and some of the bacteria are removed to prevent overcrowding, bacterial replication will continue indefinitely at exactly the same rate. When individual paramecia are placed in culture under exactly the same conditions, they at first behave in a similar fashion. They begin dividing, although it takes longer for paramecia to replicate, simply because of their size; there is a great deal more to reproduce at each cell division. They divide asexually, by fission, just like bacteria. And like bacteria, the two daughter cells resulting from asexual fission are identical in every way, including genetically. But at some point, after a hundred or so cell divisions, even if the medium is replenished and the paramecia are thinned out periodically, the initial growth rate slows. The cells change shape, and their internal chemistry changes in ways that foreshadow the changes we see in our own cells as we age. The best guess is that these changes are triggered by cumulative damage to DNA in the macronucleus. Eventually, after 200 or so cell divisions, the cells stop replicating altogether, and then they die. This is a classic example of programmed cell death.

But this slow slide through replicative senescence to death can be completely reversed if the paramecia have sex. Sex in reproduction means simply mixing together the DNA from two genetically different individuals, repairing it and recombining it to make slightly different combinations of genes than had existed in the two parental cells. These new genetic combinations are then tested in the environment for any possible advantages to the organism bearing them; those that are advantageous eventually spread throughout the breeding population; those that fail simply disappear. When paramecia multiply in culture by simple fission, like the bacteria do, they do not use sex in their reproduction. Both the macronuclear and micronuclear DNA are replicated at cell division, the replicate copies being passed into two daughter cells without modification. But when two paramecia decide to have sex (in a process called conjugation), a different procedure is followed. The two conjugating cells make extra copies of their micronuclei, repair the DNA in them, and exchange copies with each other. They then combine their own micronuclear DNA with the micronuclear DNA received from the conjugating partner, to create an entirely new and genetically unique micronucleus.

It is these new genetic combinations that must be tested against environmental challenges to determine whether they confer any advantage for survival or future reproduction; it is these new combinations of DNA upon which evolution, through natural selection, will act. But it is not the micronuclear DNA that must be tested against the environment; it is the DNA actually used to operate the cell—the macronuclear DNA. So once the new micronucleus is formed, the old macronucleus must be destroyed; a new one is then generated from the newly recombined DNA in the micronucleus. Once this has been accomplished, the sexually regenerated cells are set free to test themselves in the real world.

Very recently it was discovered that the death of the macronucleus in paramecia that have just had sex is essentially identical to the destruction of nuclei in mammalian cells undergoing apoptosis. The DNA is fragmented into millions of useless pieces. The apoptotic death of the macronucleus in early organisms such as paramecia likely represents the evolutionary beginnings of apoptotic cell death in eukaryotes. Apoptosis of the macronucleus in connection with sexual rejuvenation obviously does not lead to death of the cell, but as we will see in a moment, when carried forward into multicellular animals that is precisely what apoptosis does. Whether or not apoptotic destruction is involved in the programmed cell death that finally comes at the end of replicative senescence in these paramecia is not clear at present, although it seems very likely to be the case.

So senescence and compulsory death did appear at a specific point in evolution, and they did have to be selected and fixed as stable traits in those species in which they evolved. There was no other choice for paramecia or for any of the other protists in which it occurs, once sex was used to create new genetic combinations. And in a very real sense, the death of the macronucleus in paramecia predicts our own corporeal deaths. Paramecia had created macronuclei to deal with the challenge of size, and they had become about as large as single cells can be. The next major development in the evolutionary theme of ever-greater size was for organisms to become multicellular. Once this happened, the micronuclear (reproductive) DNA was partitioned off into germ cells; the functional equivalent of the macronuclear DNA came to occupy all the other cells of the body—the somatic cells. Like the micronuclear DNA, germ-cell DNA is recombined with the DNA of another individual during reproduction, and the new genetic combinations are passed on to the next generation. This kind of DNA is, in effect, immortal. As in paramecia, germ-cell DNA is not used to operate the resulting organism—that is the task of the somatic DNA. And just as with the macronucleus of paramecia, the old somatic DNA of multicellular eukaryotes must be destroyed once reproduction has occurred. Unfortunately, that somatic DNA, housed now in somatic cells rather than a macronucleus, is us.

Another single-cell eukaryote in which replicative senescence can be readily detected is the simple yeast *Saccharomyces cerevisiae*, used in baking and in brewing alcoholic beverages. Yeast are not protists, like the paramecia. They belong to a separate and evolutionarily slightly more advanced kingdom, the *Fungi*. These cells reproduce by a process called budding. As with simple fission in prokaryotes, one yeast cell gives rise to two; the DNA is first doubled, and one copy is passed into the daughter cell emerging as a bud from the mother's cell wall. The other copy is retained by the mother cell.

Unlike true fission as used by bacteria and paramecia, the two cells resulting from budding are not otherwise equal. Yeast cells are quite large, and the cells emerging from a budding event can be segregated and followed separately. The individual identity of the cell in which budding originates (the mother cell) is preserved when the process is finished; the product of budding is not two identical daughter cells, but a mother and a daughter. And the mother is older than before budding began. In fact, these yeast cells have a lifespan that is defined in terms of the number of buddings they can undergo, rather than a fixed period of days or months. In *Saccharomyces*, the average lifespan is about twenty-five budding events, although there is considerable variation around this average. By manipulating growth conditions to either speed up or slow down the budding process, the calendar lifespan of a yeast cell can be shortened or lengthened, accordingly. Yeast are among those cells that can form spores, or that can be stored frozen, without altering the set number of replications the cells undergo to define a lifetime.

As a mother yeast cell progresses through its lifespan, it undergoes changes that readily distinguish it from its daughters. Each time a cell gives rise to a daughter, a small scar is created on the surface at the point where the budding event took place. Over time, as much as 50 percent of the cell surface may be covered by these "birth scars." With each round of cell replication, the cell also becomes slightly larger; about 20 percent in volume with each cell cycle. There are also progressive, subtle changes in a specialized compartment of the nucleus called the nucleolus of the mother cell that are not transmitted to the daughter. And finally, the time to complete a budding event gradually increases with each succeeding event. A very young yeast cell requires about sixty minutes to produce a daughter by budding; at the very end of its lifespan, the same cell may require as long as six hours to reproduce. The daughter cells produced from a budding event will experience the same total lifespan as the mother; the aging clock in the daughter cell is essentially reset to zero. But at some point these daughters, too, will senesce; they will undergo the same internal changes, slow down, stop dividing, and die via programmed cell death. This gradual slide through reduced metabolic activity toward arrested cell division and death represents another expression of replicative senescence.

An interesting and fundamentally important feature of replicative senescence in *Saccharomyces* is that it is a dominant trait. For example, when an older cell gives rise to a daughter by budding, the daughter will actually divide somewhat slowly for one or two cell divisions, at the rate of the mother, before rebounding to the more rapid replication rate of a younger cell. Daughters of younger mothers, on the other hand, begin reproducing rapidly immediately after separation from the mother. Moreover, if a younger cell is mated with an older cell, the resulting hybrid will have a remaining lifespan dictated by the older partner, not the younger (or some intermediate value.) This has given rise to the notion that aging in these cells is regulated by a diffusable substance resident in the cells' cytoplasm. Newly generated daughters are apparently able to neutralize the effect of this substance, whereas older cells (including those that engage in mating) cannot. We will examine the genes that may code for such factors in a later chapter on the genetic control of replicative senescence.

So in yeast, as in paramecia, we see the existence of senescence, again in the form of replicative senescence. There is no macronucleus in yeast, necessitating apoptotic destruction in connection with reproduction, but it is clear that yeast are capable of apoptosis, and it is very likely that the programmed death ultimately resulting from senescence is apoptotic. In unicellular eukaryotes such as yeast and paramecia, death of the cell is of course equivalent to death of the organism. But in multicellular animals, this is not necessarily true. As we have seen, in higher eukaryotes apoptosis is used largely in the process of shaping organs and tissues during embryonic development. The death of enough cells of key types in an adult organism—heart or brain cells, for example—could lead quickly to death of the entire individual. But the more likely outcome of cumulative apoptotic cell death is a gradual deterioration of the various organs and tissues that are composed of these cells, contributing to the pathologies of aging that ultimately result in death of the organism through accident or from "natural causes." Remarkably, the genes and proteins involved in apoptosis in the unicellular eukaryotes, in those cases where they have been identified, are very similar to the genes and proteins used for these same purposes in higher eukaryotes, including humans. It would seem that the genetic programs underlying senescence and programmed cell death apppeared very early in eukaryotic evolution, and have been highly conserved throughout some three billion years of subsequent evolution.

Replicative Senescence in Higher Animals

The replicative senescence seen in yeast and paramecia can also be observed in almost all eukaryotic cells, including those of humans and other higher animals, although for many years this was overlooked because of a misinterpreted experiment. In the early 1900s Alexis Carrel, a French physician-scientist working in the United States, claimed to have grown a single line of chicken embryo fibroblasts continuously in culture for over thirty years. Fibroblasts are the component cells of connective tissue, found ubiquitously throughout the tissues and organs of most birds and mammals. Fibroblasts are among the few cells of the body that will readily undergo replication outside the body. The cultures were kept at roughly the body temperature of a living chicken, and subdivided frequently to prevent overcrowding. Fresh nutrients were provided at each subdivision. Carrel's experiments provided a major stimulus to the growth and study of cells in vitro. Over the next fifty years conditions for growing many different types of cells were gradually improved; in vitro cell culture would prove key to resolving many important questions about cell biology, especially in higher animals.

But perhaps the most fundamental impact of Carrel's finding was on our views of senescence, an incorrect view that unfortunately lasted over forty years. The implication of Carrel's work was that aging and death were in a sense in vivo ("in life," i.e., in the body) artifacts; the idea developed that individual cells are basically immortal, but something in the in vivo environment condemns them to mortality. Individual cells taken from the embryos were living well beyond the maximum lifespan of even the best-kept chickens. Moreover, the effective biomass generated from a few of Carrel's fibroblasts, if all of the subdivisions had been fully maintained (most were simply thrown away) would have been equivalent to millions of chickens within a year or so. Thus the normal aging and death of animals came to be viewed as a program imposed on cells that, if left on their own, would neither age nor die. But clearly this program was not inherent in the cells themselves; it had to be imposed by events taking place inside the body. It followed that understanding and controlling senescence and death should revolve around identifying these extracellular factors or agents present in the body that rendered the cells mortal. The unfortunate result of this idea was that for half a century all aging research was carried out only in whole organisms or on populations. Important insights that would come from studying senescence in cells would be delayed for many years.

Carrel's interpretation of cellular senescence and death was called into question and ultimately refuted by an elegant series of experiments begun in the 1960s by Leonard Hayflick and his colleague Paul Moorhead working at the Wistar Institute in Philadelphia. (Hayflick eventually moved to Stanford University in California.) Hayflick found that when human embryonic fibroblasts were cultured in vitro, they did not replicate indefinitely as Carrel had claimed, but seemed to be limited to a total of about fifty to sixty cell divisions. The same was found to be true of fibroblasts from a wide range of animal sources, including chickens, and ultimately of other cell types as well. It was very difficult for Hayflick and his colleagues to have their results accepted in the beginning. Everyone assumed these younger and less experienced researchers were simply careless, or lacking in some crucial knowledge of how to do cell culture. Others had also failed to confirm Carrel's claims, but Carrel and his associates always pointed out that great care had to be taken to maintain these delicate cells in vitro over long periods of time; not just anyone could do it. So for many years the failures of others were simply ignored in favor of Carrel's more intriguing hypothesis.

Hayflick and Moorhead, however, were incredibly persistent, and quite ingenious in their experimental designs. One elegant demonstration of their thesis came from mixing old cells taken from males with young cells collected from a female. The identity of the cells involved could readily be established by looking at the chromosomal makeup, which is distinct for the two sexes. After a period of time, the only cells dividing in the mixed cultures were from the female donor; all of the male cells had stopped growing. This experiment provided powerful evidence that the replicative senescence they were observing was real, and was an innate property of the cells themselves, rather than an artifact of their culturing methods. Soon others began to follow their lead, and before too much longer other scientists became confident in their own failures to reproduce Carrel's findings. (This period of exciting research history is admirably recounted by Hayflick himself in his book, *How and Why We Age* (1994).) It turned out that some of the materials used by Carrel to feed his chicken fibroblast cultures were themselves probably contaminated with fresh chicken embryo cells. Rather than simply feeding his cultures once a week, he was reseeding them with young, vigorous new cells!

The new view, promulgated by Hayflick over many years of fruitful investigations which he continued at Stanford, is that fibroblasts (and in fact virtually every eukaryotic cell that has been looked at) display a definite replicative senescence. If removed from a rapidly growing in vivo source like an embryo, and cultured in vitro, they will grow vigorously at first, with a relatively short cell-cycle time (the time required to undergo one complete round of cell replication). However, after a certain number of cycles, the cells become noticeably larger and begin to divide more slowly, very much like paramecia or yeast; fibroblasts also appear to have "life clocks" based on a set number of cell divisions, rather than on standard calendar time. If embryonic fibroblasts are frozen partway through their set number of cycles, then thawed and placed back into culture, they will continue toward completion of their program just as though nothing had happened, even though they may have been stored in the frozen state for many years. Moreover, fibroblasts harvested from "middle-aged" individuals will undergo a proportionally reduced number of cell cycles in vitro; cells from very old individuals will divide only a few times before stopping. Fibroblasts harvested from the same individual may have differing replicative lifespans in vitro: Cells taken from skin in a region of the body normally protected from sun will undergo more divisions in vitro than cells from a region receiving intense sun exposure.

Hayflick proposed that the replicative behavior of fibroblasts in vitro reflected some aspect of the aging process in vivo, and to a first approximation, this is generally accepted by everyone who studies aging. Not all cells in a mature organism continue to divide throughout life, so completing a set number of cell cycles cannot be a general basis for cellular or organismal senescence; Hayflick himself never claimed this. What is perhaps more likely is that the senescent processes leading to the deterioration of cellular functions generally, in the in vivo setting, affect cell division in those cells that divide in vitro. Replicative failure is thus more likely a reflection of, rather than a primary cause of, senescence. Support for this notion comes from the finding that biochemical changes occurring within fibroblasts dividing in vitro correspond closely to the changes that occur within cells of the body as they age in vivo, whether they divide or not. Interestingly, replicative senescence is also echoed in maximum lifespan, in that the number of in vitro replications characterizing the fibroblasts from a given species correlates directly with its maximum lifespan. Mouse or rat embryo fibroblasts, for example, divide only about a dozen times; humans, as we have noted, about fifty; and the Galapagos turtle, about 120 times. This is one of the strongest arguments that replicative senescence is in some way tied into the normal aging process.

What happens to fibroblasts at the end of their "life" in vitro is really not known. Despite a few claims to the contrary, there is ample evidence they do not die, at least not as an immediate consequence of the loss of the ability to divide. They simply lie idly in their culture dishes, continuing to make RNA and proteins, responding to many signals from the outside with an appropriate response—except for signals to begin replicating. At this stage they are behaving pretty much like cells removed from older people in terms of what they can and cannot do. It seems unlikely that cells that age naturally in culture and enter senescence are truly immortal, but unfortunately no one has yet followed them out in time to see whether and how they die. This is an experiment that should be done to complete the story of replicative senescence in vitro.

Programmed cell death in multicellular animals has become more complex in humans and other multicellular animals than it was in the early eukaryotes, and also has found other uses such as the shaping of body parts during mammalian embryogenesis. But this cell death program has also been maintained over enormous periods of evolutionary time, and has been incorporated as one element of a larger scheme— senescence—for assuring the eventual death of all eukaryotic organisms. The genes underlying programmed cell death have been maintained rigorously since its appearance in the earliest eukaryotes. We can think of this scheme as one part of the "programmed death" of the organism, but we must define our terms carefully. Clearly there is no defined program, in the sense of a series of steps that are executed in a set sequence, eventually culminating in death of an organism. Rather, a collection of senescence-inducing mechanisms, based on cellular senescence and leading to the eventual extinction of the somatic organism, has become part of the eukaryotic heritage. A very large proportion of these mechanisms were in fact already in place in the earliest single-cell eukaryotic organisms.

Nonreplicative Senescence in Eukaryotic Cells

Not all cells divide; in fact, aside from cells lining the intestines, skin cells, bone marrow cells, and a few other examples, most cells in adult organisms do not divide most of the time. Some, such as mature muscle and nerve cells, may never divide. The relevance of replicative senescence to such cells is not immediately obvious. So what happens to nondividing cells as they grow old?

A great many biochemical and morphological changes have been recorded in aging, nondividing cells, and although at least some of them seem potentially harmful, it must be admitted that the significance of most of these changes is not clear. We know, for example, that cells tend to lose water as they age, probably reflecting an alteration in the function of the membrane pumps discussed earlier. This cellular dehydration in turn affects how the organism looks; newborn infants are about 80 percent water, whereas water is less than 50 percent of the body mass of a wizened, older individual.

As they age, cells tend to accumulate materials not found in younger cells. These are often thought of as accumulated biochemical "trash," but there is no real basis for such an assumption. One of the most common of these materials is something called lipofuscin, or "age pigment" because of its universal distribution in older people. (These are not the pigments that accumulate in skin, but rather within cells of most of the major internal organs, particularly the nervous system.) Lipofuscin is found in intracellular granules, and in very old individuals these granules may appear to be crowding out cellular organelles and threatening their functional integrity. The major component of lipofuscin is fat, and in particular fat that has been oxidatively damaged. Fats (or lipids) are also a major component of both internal and external cell membranes; these lipids also become oxidized with age which results in increased rigidity and reduced functionality. Damage of cellular components by oxidative by-products of metabolism is a major source of cellular degeneration in aging. Oxidation of proteins in the lens and capsule of the eye is a major cause of cataracts, for example. The gradual oxidative degradation of mitochondria, the energy-producing organelles of the cell, is also thought to be a major element in cellular senescence.

One of the potentially most damaging changes that can occur within a cell as it ages is mutation of the DNA. This can be caused by toxic oxidative wastes generated within the cell, or by radiation impinging on those cells that lie close to the surface of the body. Damage to DNA by ultraviolet components of sunlight is a major factor in aging of the skin, and a major cause of skin cancer. Cells are equipped to repair DNA damage, but this ability falls off with age, and the resulting alterations in DNA, including loss of gene function, is thought to be a major cause of senescence in both dividing and non-dividing cells.

Many cells alter their secretions as they age, and the materials secreted can impair the ability of the organism as a whole to function. Proteins categorized generically as amyloids are secreted by a number of cells scattered throughout the body. Once outside the cell, they condense into compacted amyloid fibrils, which are a common finding in Alzheimer's disease, as well as in heart tissue where they can contribute to congestive heart failure. Collagen is secreted by many cell types in the body, and forms the basic tissue matrix in which cells live. As cells age, the collagen they secrete changes in nature, becoming more rigid, even brittle. Because collagen is so widespread in the body, the general degradation of this "extracellular matrix" is thought by many to be a major impediment to efficient functioning of many organs, and a major contributor to overall senescence.

Any or all of the above cellular changes could contribute significantly to the overall senescence of the organism. The array of changes in an organism resulting from senescence—the "aging phenotype"—is enormous and complex; the changes for humans listed in Table 1.1 are just the tip of the iceberg. At the cellular level, the total number of changes is more limited, and the same changes are observed in virtually all eukaryotes as they senesce, whether the cells in question are replicating or not. The challenge for the biogerontologist is not only to untangle the causes of organismal senescence from one another, but to try to understand how they relate to underlying causes of cellular senescence. And at the cellular level, where senescence is still multifaceted, the task will be to determine which causes of senescence are truly primary, and to understand their genetic and molecular basis. Then, and only then, will we truly understand the aging process. This investigation is well under way, and what we have learned so far is described in the remainder of this book.

3

The Evolution of Senescence and Death

A great many discussions about the evolution of senescence begin with the question of <u>how senescence could have evolved</u> in the first place. This question has long puzzled some of the best thinkers in evolutionary biology and genetics. Senescence as we understand it in eukaryotes does not exist, or at least has never been reliably detected, in prokaryotic organisms. It seems to have evolved very early in eukaryotic history, close in time to their emergence from the prokaryotes and to the beginning of the use of sex in reproduction.

From our understanding of the principles of evolution and natural selection, it is easy to imagine how traits like increased physical vigor, better eyesight, or brighter plumage for attracting mates—traits that would increase reproductive fitness or prolong the reproductive lifespan of an individual organism—could arise within, and eventually come to dominate, a breeding population. It is less obvious how something like senescence—which severely impairs an organism's ability to function in its natural environment—could have been positively selected under these same rules. As individuals get older, their ability to find mates, reproduce, and, where necessary, care for offspring are all seriously impaired by aging. So how could genetic variants promoting aging ever have been selected in evolution?

This mystery is compounded by the fact that, in the wild, most animals do not live long enough to experience serious aging. They die from disease or predation long before they become noticeably old; for most species, elderly individuals can be found only in zoos or laboratories. That means that the very thing natural selection is supposed to act upon rarely ever shows up in nature. Yet, if kept in zoos or labs, animals definitely do age. But where did the genes responsible for aging come from?

To get around these problems, some of the early evolutionary theorists proposed that certain traits may be selected for in evolution that are contrary to the interests of the individual, as long as they benefit the species to which the individual belongs. It was proposed that as long as such traits ultimately enhanced the ability of members of the species to pass on their genes, the interests of the individual would be served (albeit as part of a larger group), and thus such a mechanism would be consistent with evolution via natural selection.

The problem with such "group selectionist" theories is that there is simply no known mechanism whereby they could actually work. As we will discuss in more detail in a moment, variants of existing genes arise within an individual organism. They either allow that individual to breed more effectively, or they don't. If they do, the new variants can, as a result of enhanced breeding efficiency of the "founding" individual and its offspring, over many generations come to be carried by a significant number of other individuals in the species. If the new gene confers no particular reproductive advantage, it may linger for awhile, but will be unlikely to spread very far into the rest of the species. If the new gene decreases reproductive efficiency, it will quickly disappear. This is the only basis on which natural selection can operate. There is simply no way to imagine how a gene arising in an individual could be acted on by natural selection *on behalf of a species as a whole*. There is no way for nature to anticipate, at the point in time when a new genetic variant arises, possible future advantages a gene might have for the entire species. Yet a decision about the value of the new variant must be made at the time that it arises. And this decision can be made only

in terms of the individual in which it arises, or that individual's immediate offspring. Thus, while there exist several examples of genes that
would seem to confer benefits to the species rather than the individual, group selection as an explanation of their existence has been abandoned by all serious evolutionists for lack of a reasonable mechanism
to explain it.

Genes, Mutations, and Evolution

Before launching into a discussion of the evolution of senescence, let's take a brief moment to discuss the nature of genes, genetic
mutations, and natural selection, which are the working components
of evolution. We will discuss these topics here only in the broadest outlines; more detailed explanations will be provided in connection with
specific examples as they arise. Genes are stretches of DNA that direct
the production of proteins in a cell. Humans have approximately
100,000 genes distributed over twenty-three pairs of chromosomes
stored in the nucleus of each cell in the body. This collection of genes
in its entirety is referred to as the genome. Every aspect of a cell's life
history is directed by proteins synthesized according to the instructions
contained in genes. A set of genes sufficient to provide all the proteins
needed for the construction and operation of a complete organism is
contained in the genome copies stored in each cell. When an organism reproduces, it transmits a copy of its genome to its offspring
through the special subset of cells known as germ cells (sperm and ova
in humans). The remaining cells of the body—the somatic cells—are
not involved directly in reproduction, but rather serve to support the
ability of the germ cells to transmit genes to the next generation.

Mutations are alterations in DNA that change the nature of genes
and thus of the proteins produced. All eukaryotic organisms have two
copies of each gene, one inherited from the father, and one from the
mother, the state referred to as diploidy. For almost all genes, there are
slightly different variants, created by mutation and scattered throughout the population. By definition, all of these variants are functional;
the minor changes they represent create a spectrum of functional proteins, some better than others, but all within a range compatible with
supporting life. These variants of genes are called alleles. The particular collection of alleles within the genome of any individual member

of a species is defined as that individual's genotype. The number of different possible combinations—genotypes—is of course enormous, and so virtually every member of a species (except for genetically identical twins) will have a different genotype. All members will have the same set of genes; they will just have different combinations of alleles of those genes. The observable differences in characteristics dictated by the differing alleles distributed throughout a species are referred to as phenotypes—height or eye color, for example.

New alleles arise by the process of mutation, slight changes in DNA coding sequences that arise during evolution. These changes can occur through damage to the DNA or through errors made in copying the DNA during cellular replication. If a new allele is either neutral or beneficial to the reproductive efficiency of the individual in which it arises, it may, as just discussed, find its way into some portion of the rest of the species. Any mutation that results in decreased reproductive efficiency will disappear from the population, since it will be difficult to pass on to succeeding generations. The consequences of such mutations are in one sense catastrophic, since all of the other genes in the genome of that individual also disappear.

For organisms that exist on the earth today, which are the products of millions of years of evolutionary experimentation through mutation and natural selection, most new mutations are neutral or harmful, meaning the protein encoded by the altered gene will not function better than the unmutated form, and may not work as well. If the alteration is reproductively lethal, the mutation will disappear. If the mutation is functionally neutral, or maybe even slightly less efficient than the gene in which it arose, it may be kept within a species as a minor allele. However, on rare occasions, a mutation may actually improve the function of a given protein, and in so doing improve the ability of organisms in which the mutation is expressed to cope with their environment. If this results in increased reproductive efficiency, the new allele will likely be "fixed" in the species through natural selection; that is, it will come to be expressed by a significant portion of its members.

Mutations can occur either in somatic cells or in germ cells. Should a mutation occur in a somatic cell, in most cases the mutation, even if harmful, will have little effect, because that cell is just one cell out of billions that make up the organism. If that somatic cell divides during its lifetime to give rise to other cells, then the progeny of that somatic cell will inherit the mutation and be similarly affected. But cell replication in most organs and tissues is relatively rare, so the effects of somatic mutations are usually quite limited. An obvious exception, of course, are those mutations that cause normal somatic cells to become cancerous.

Mutations in germ cells differ in two important ways from somatic cell mutations. First, they are much more frequent; in fact, there are special mechanisms in germ cells that encourage alteration of the DNA during replication to create new genetic possibilities. Second, germ cells are involved in the formation of an entire new organism; thus a mutation in a germ cell will show up in every single cell of subsequent offspring, including those offspring's own germ cells. These mutations will be acted upon by the forces of natural selection to weed out from the breeding population those that affect the organism negatively, and to retain those that affect the organism positively. Again, the genes of those organisms that are able to reproduce most efficiently will become established within a breeding population, and perhaps come to dominate in that population. The genes of those organisms that reproduce less effectively will diminish in the breeding population, and likely disappear.

The range of genetic traits that can affect reproduction is enormous. In fact, from a fundamental evolutionary point of view, every single molecule composing an organism, whether in somatic cells or germ cells, serves only one single purpose: maximization of the ability of the organism to pass its genes on to the next generation. Genes regulating the ability to see or to smell, to move or to think, as well as to identify a mate, produce germ cells, and engage in actual reproduction—all of these are dedicated to helping the organism reproduce its genome and pass it on to its offspring. Natural selection has no other basis for "decision making" than the impact of natural variation—mutations—on the survival and reproduction of genes. It is worth remembering that evolution is not the "purpose" of natural selection. Natural selection ultimately adheres to the same principles of thermodynamics that govern all other activities in the physical universe; evolution is simply an epiphenomenon perceived by humans.

Nonevolutionary Theories of Senescence

Prior to the establishment and general acceptance of Darwin's principles of evolution, and the subsequent realization that heredity is controlled by genes, aging was viewed largely as a process of mechanical degradation. August Weismann addressed this issue in a series of influential lectures in the 1880s. Weismann recognized the value of death in "making room" for the next generation, freeing up resources for that generation's own reproductive activities. The problem with this idea, of course, is that we have no idea how mutations working toward such an abstract goal would be selected in evolution. Nevertheless, Weismann imagined that aging and death probably result simply from wearing out of parts of the organism, like many mechanical devices known at the time.

Examples of mechanical wear of animal parts certainly do exist. The teeth in animals such as horses wear down noticeably with age, and are not replaced; "failures" of this type could easily contribute to death. But in fact, most mechanical wear in animal tissues and organs is repairable, making comparisons with truly mechanical devices specious. Moreover, if we are to interpret senescence in animals in terms of senescence at the cellular level, we would want to specify precisely which cellular or subcellular components would "wear out" over time in a manner that could contribute to senescence of the whole organism.

The most likely molecular candidate for mechanical wear at a cellular level would be proteins, and a great deal of energy has gone into investigating whether proteins wear out in a way and with a timing that would help explain organismal senescence. Proteins participate in two main ways in the life of a cell. First, they are involved in the physical structure of the cell, for example, as components of cell membranes that are found not only at the surface of the cell, but folded up throughout the cell in the form of the organelles, small organ-like structures that perform various physiological tasks within the cell. Proteins are also the major structural element of the cytoskeleton—stiff, rod-like structures that help the cell maintain its three-dimensional shape, participate in the cell's movements from one place to another, or anchor the cell in a fixed position within the body.

In addition to their structural roles, proteins are also the major functional elements of the cell, in the form of enzymes. There are literally hundreds of different enzymes in each cell, each one catalyzing a different step in the multistep breakdown of food and construction from the resulting materials of the hundreds of different structural and functional molecules needed by the cell. Only proteins are directly encoded in DNA; every other molecule in the cell—carbohydrates, fats, even the DNA itself—is synthesized from the breakdown products of food (or intracellular waste products) in a series of enzyme-catalyzed reactions. The regulation of DNA expression within a cell, and the copying of DNA into messages that can be read by the cell, are also carried out by proteins. Enzymes are involved in the generation of energy in the cell, supplying the fuel that drives each of the cell's metabolic activities, including operation of the membrane pumps that keep water out of the cell, and maintain the cell's proper ionic balance with respect to the extracellular environment. Many of the products exported by cells, hormones like insulin, for example, or the globins involved in oxygen transport, are also proteins.

Because of the importance of proteins in the life of the cell, it is certainly easy to imagine that damage accumulating over time to cellular proteins could contribute to the gradual breakdown of cellular function. In the 1960s it was proposed that, particularly because of the role of proteins in regulating and reading DNA, even slight changes in the structure or function of proteins over time could have catastrophic consequences for the cell, perhaps causing changes that express themselves as aging. This hypothesis was put forward in a persuasive way, and stimulated numerous experiments that are still going on in various laboratories.

The results have not been particularly encouraging. Proteins from older cells do not appear to be deformed or riddled with errors, although some slight differences are apparent in comparisons with younger cells. Defective proteins cannot be repaired, but cells are equipped with machinery to weed out and dispose of damaged or incorrectly made proteins, and this procedure seems still to be working well in older cells. Proteins can be modified by oxidation, or by the nonspecific addition of sugar molecules (glycation), and this can result in loss of function, but it is not clear that this is involved in normal cellular senescence.

The problem is that we do not really know what degree of protein damage would lead to senescent changes within a cell. Shorter-lived proteins such as enzymes are replaced frequently within the cell, and would have little opportunity to accumulate lethal errors. Although accumulation of errors in the more stable and longer lasting structural proteins could conceivably contribute to aging, it must be admitted that compelling evidence for a general "wearing out" of nonrepairable molecules as a general explanation for senescence has not been gathered, and most researchers are looking elsewhere for the solution to the aging problem. One of the most telling arguments against the wearing out of proteins as an explanation of senescence, in view of their nonrepairability, is that mice and humans, although composed of proteins that are extremely similar at a chemical level, have both average and maximal lifespans differing by a factor of 30 or more.

On the other hand, many other components of a cell are in fact repairable, through the action of the enzymes. Damage to lipid structures and to complex carbohydrates (sugars and starches) are subject to enzymatic detection, degradation, and repair. Ongoing repair of these molecules is vital to the overall health of the cells. Perhaps most important, in terms of aging, is the detection and repair of damage to DNA. The integrity of the DNA is absolutely vital to the integrity of the cell, which is in turn the foundation of fitness and vitality of the organism. Prior to reproductive maturity, a great deal of energy is spent examining and repairing DNA, particularly in cells that divide. Once the organism is reproductively mature, damage to DNA continues to accrue, but less and less effort is expended in repairing it. This balance between damage and repair of DNA is one of the most important aspects of cellular senescence, and is a theme to which we will return repeatedly in the following chapters.

Evolutionary Theories of Senescence

As our knowledge of genetics began to expand in the early years of the twentieth century, the realization gradually developed that senescence and maximum lifespan are likely to be controlled by hereditary factors. The evidence for this was certainly, at the time, indirect. It depended mostly on the observation that maximum lifespan for a given species is relatively constant for that species, and thus apparently inherited. The lifespan for two different species living in the same ecological niche can easily differ by a factor of ten or more, confirming that maxium lifespan is genetically regulated, and not entirely a consequence of environmental factors. To the extent that maximum lifespan is heritable and stable from generation to generation, and intimately tied to the timing of the onset of senescence, it was assumed lifespan and senescence would ultimately turn out to be governed by genes.

Among the earlier attempts to incorporate emerging concepts of genetics into an evolutionary basis for senescence and lifespan was the mutational accumulation theory based on the thinking of the British scientists J. B. S. Haldane in the 1940s and Peter Medawar in the 1950s. The basic idea developed by these two thinkers was that genetic mutations harmful to the organism, such as those causing senescence and physiological degeneration (senescence effector genes), would be strongly selected against in nature if the mutations came into play in an organism prior to reproductive maturity. To the extent that these mutations interfere with an organism's ability to succeed reproductively, they will not become established as alleles within the breeding population.

On the other hand, potentially harmful mutations that are not expressed until later in life, after the individual has had an adequate opportunity to reproduce, would not be selected against and could survive within the population. They would have already been passed on to the next generation before their negative effects came into play. Examples of such senescence effector genes could include some of those that predispose to certain hereditary forms of cancer, Huntington's disease, or Alzheimer's disease. These diseases are all caused by mutated forms of genes that are inherited and passed on to the next generation. However, the effects of such mutations are generally not expressed until relatively late in life, when they certainly contribute to the overall pattern of senescence seen in at least some humans.

Medawar was one of the first to point out that our ability to observe senescence in animals is in a sense an artifact, first made visible largely through domestication of animals by humans some 10,000 years ago; only when animals were nourished and protected from predators by farmers did their inherent ability to age become obvious. An interesting possibility also discussed by Medawar is that senescence effector genes may be held in check early in life by special senescence repressor genes. Senescence, on those rare occasions when it is actually expressed, would correlate with the turn-off of these repressor genes later in life, allowing the harmful genes to be expressed. It is easy to see how genes of this type might be selected for in evolution, since they would play a positive role in fostering reproduction. Although arguments of a theoretical nature have been expressed against this notion by some evolutionists, we will see shortly that a version of this idea is coming back into favor with many molecular biologists.

The general theoretical approach introduced by Haldane and Medawar was refined and extended by George Williams in a classic paper published in 1957. Like others before him, Williams assumed that senescence per se could not be positively selected for in evolution in any direct way. He also assumed that evolution and natural selection would not operate on traits expressed only in post-reproductive individuals; such individuals are, for all practical purposes, invisible to evolution. Williams proposed that some genetic alterations (alleles) positively selected during evolution on the basis of increasing early survival or improving reproductive efficiency may have harmful effects once the reproductive period has peaked. Because the advantages in terms of reproduction are so important, they outweigh the harmful effects of these senescence effector genes in the post-reproductive period, and the gene becomes fixed in the population. In common with Medawar's proposal, senescence genes are viewed as things not positively selected *for* in evolution, but rather negative by-products, not selected *against*, of more positive traits.

Williams made a great point of linking a negative genetic effect (senescence) with the selection of genes directly involved with reproduction, but this linkage is in a sense specious because, as stated earlier, evolution operates only on traits that affect reproductive efficiency; there is no other basis for natural selection. Thus any biological trait positively selected for could secondarily contribute to senescence, as long as expression of its negative effect is delayed until reproductive maturity.

Quite apart from his speculations on the evolutionary origin of genes responsible for senescence, Williams also made a series of important predictions about how reproductive timing and accidental death rates should influence fecundity, senescence, and lifespan. By and large these predictions, which have stimulated a great deal of fruitful aging research in the past four decades, are not dependent on his ideas about the origins of senescence-promoting genes. Most of the early attempts to test the validity of Williams's ideas were directed to those aspects dealing with the interactions between senescence and species mortality rates, or between senescence and reproductive maturity and fecundity. Such studies, which relied mostly on classical transmission and population genetics, have largely validated Williams's predictions.

The disposable soma theory of the evolution of senescence, formulated mostly by T. B. L. Kirkwood and his associates, and the optimality theory of aging as defined by Partridge and Barton, approach the problem from the point of view of allocation of environmental resources between reproduction and maintenance of the soma (the body of the organism exclusive of the germ cells). Particularly in situations where resources are scarce, investment of these resources in one activity (e.g., maintaining individuals beyond their breeding years) is done at the expense of other activities (e.g., reproduction). Presumably maintenance of organisms into old age would entail not simply maintenance of some minimal metabolic rate, but also investment of energy in repairing accumulated molecular and genetic damage accumulated over time. Failure to make such an investment allows this damage to take its toll, and manifests as senescence.

Mathematical equations employed in ecological studies were used to show that investment of resources in the building of an organism that would survive longer than its expected survival in the wild would be useless in terms of evolutionary advantage. What these equations basically predict is that animals with high rates of accidental death from the natural environment will have shorter maximal lifespans even when measured in a highly protected environment. This turns out to be true, or at least consistent with the limited number of observations that have been made on natural populations. Thus it would make little sense to invest scarce resources into building an organism that would last too much longer than the average natural lifespan; beyond this point the "soma" is better disposed of than maintained.

The value of evolutionary theories of senescence and death is that they remind us constantly that our interpretations of experimental data relating to these phenomena cannot exist in a vacuum, but must be consistent with what we understand about the origin and evolution of all biological phenomena. Since further experimentation is always based on interpretations of previous experimental results, restrictions placed on these interpretations help guide further research. The theories in turn are of course subject to modification as additional data are gathered. Mutational theories drive the experimenter to define genes whose mutation may be involved in senescence. The disposable soma and other optimality theories do not suggest underlying mechanisms that could be directly tested, but they provide useful yardsticks against which mechanistic experiments can be judged. As we will see in later chapters, with the exception of speculations on the origin of senescence effector and senescence repressor genes, the evolutionary theories developed so far are in fact consistent with most of the data collected in the past several decades, suggesting they may be essentially correct, at least in broad outline.

Experimental Manipulation of Senescence and Lifespan

Like all good scientific hypotheses, most of the theoretical models for the evolution of senescence make several clear predictions that ought to be subject to experimental validation. One prediction deriving from all of these hypotheses is that populations that reproduce early in their lifespan should have a relatively short maximum lifespan, and those populations reproducing later in their lifespan should have a longer lifespan. This would also be compatible with the notion implicit in these theories that interspecies variability in maximum lifespan is related to the length of time senescence is delayed in order to permit reproduction and, where appropriate, subsequent care of offspring.

In the early 1980s, two laboratories set out to test these predictions, using various strains of the common fruit fly *Drosophila melanogaster* as a model system. Drosophila (we will adopt the terminology used by Drosophila researchers and refer to them hereafter simply as "flies") have many advantages as an experimental system. The genetics and biochemistry of flies are known in more detail than almost any other multicellular eukaryotic laboratory animal. They are small and inexpensive to maintain, have a short life cycle, and breed early—two weeks post-hatching, on average; this means that experiments with very large numbers of subjects over many generations, crucial for studies of evolutionary questions, are easy to perform. On the down side, one could ask how relevant information gained in flies may be to senescence and lifespan in higher organisms, including humans. This question was addressed in a 1981 study that showed that at a cellular level, and even at the level of comparable organs, flies go through senescence-related changes that are remarkably similar to mammals. One of the amazing realizations to come out of twentieth-century biology is the remarkable uniformity of cellular processes among organisms as diverse and evolutionarily separated as humans and flies and bacteria.

The design of the aging experiments with Drosophila was quite straightforward. Flies were allowed to breed and lay eggs, but eggs for hatching were selected from increasingly later stages of the female reproductive cycle. (Flies normally undergo several rounds of mating and egg-laying.) For example, in an early study reported by Michael Rose, eggs were collected from females laying them on day 28, toward the end of the egg-laying period for most flies. These eggs were allowed to hatch, and females from this brood were mated. Eggs were again collected only at day 28, and this was repeated for several generations. Eggs were then collected that were laid on day 35 for a few generations. The egg-gathering time was gradually moved up through successive generations to 70 days, well beyond the average longevity of most unselected flies (very few normally live past fifty days.) The flies hatching at the end of these selection procedures were tested for two things: average and maximum lifespans, and the timing of reproduction.

Flies emerging from eggs laid at 70 days displayed decreased fecundity (production of offspring) early in life, compared with unselected controls, and increased fecundity later in life. The selected characteristic was stable, and bred true. The impact of selection on overall survival was quite clear; unselected flies had a mean survival time of about 33 days, while the selected flies survived an average of 43 days, an increase of roughly one-third in average lifespan. The maximum possible lifespan for this group of flies was also increased, although, because of the small numbers surviving at the very end, firm conclusions cannot be drawn from the data shown. More recent experiments with larger numbers of flies and stricter selection conditions have produced strains with double the normal average longevity, with a corresponding increase in maximum lifespan.

These experiments suggest that, as predicted by the evolutionary theories of senescence, delaying the onset of reproduction (the parameter actively selected for in these experiments) over many generations delays the onset of senescence, which is in turn associated with an increase in maximum lifespan. We assume that in these experiments, flies whose inherent genetic programs led them to reproduce (and die) at younger ages were gradually weeded from the breeding pool over time. In other words, new characteristics controlled by new genes were not being developed and fixed by natural selection; that would take many more generations than were involved in these experiments. Rather, the population was enriched for individuals already expressing natural variants of genes and gene combinations favoring prolonged lifespan—variants that were already in the natural gene pool. These would presumably be the individuals forming the tail-end slope of the curves in Figure 1.1, C, and also the ones providing the very long-term survivors in Carey's study with millions of medflies.

One of the more convincing experiments on the interaction of sexual maturation and lifespan was carried out largely in the wild, rather than in the laboratory, and involved the tiny tropical fish known as guppies. Guppies (*Poecilia reticulata*) are quite common on the island of Trinidad, just off the coast of Venezuela, where they are found in the rivers spilling down from the mountains of the Northern Range toward the sea. These rivers are very steep, and are interrupted by cascades and waterfalls, which effectively segregate guppy populations in a single river into pools of noninteracting populations. It also segregates the guppies' predators. In the lower parts of the rivers, the natural predator is the pike cichlid *Crenicichla alta*, which preys only on sexually mature guppies. Several waterfalls up in each river, the major guppy predator is the killifish *Rivulus harti*, which selectively preys on pre-reproductive guppies.

Evolutionary theories of senescence would predict that in an isolated population with a high accidental mortality rate among reproductively mature adults (downstream guppies), natural selection would favor the generation of individuals that reach sexual maturity early in life, and who invest more of their resources in early-life reproductive activity. And indeed that is what David Reznick and his colleagues, who have been studying these populations in Trinidad for nearly twenty years, have found (Table 3.1). To study the reproductive behavior of individuals produced in different predatory environments, guppies were collected from various river pools and moved to the lab-

Table 3.1. *Effect of different predatory patterns on the average lifespan of guppies in the rivers of Trinidad*

Population studied	Average age of reproductively mature fish	
	Males	Females
Lower river pools: predator *C. alta* (prefers reproductively mature guppies)	48.4 days	85.1 days
Upper river pools: predator *R. harti* (prefers pre-reproductive guppies)	56.3 days	95.0 days
Guppies transferred from lower river pools to higher pools, after five years	52.4 days	91.0 days
C. alta moved to upper river pools, after eleven years	58.2 days	92.3 days

oratory for two generations, where they were given an adequate food supply and protected from predators. Two generations is sufficient time to adapt to the new laboratory environment, but is insufficient time for any genetic changes in response to the new environment to occur. The conditions used thus allowed the investigators to observe, in the relative absence of accidental death, the breeding behavior produced by natural selection of these fish in the wild. When large numbers of individuals from several different rivers were taken into account, it was found that both males and females in the lower river populations reached sexual maturity 8–10 days earlier than fish bred in the upper river pools, where breeding adults were the targets of the natural predator. In terms of the human reproductive lifespan, this would be equivalent to achieving sexual maturity at age 9–10, versus the normal 12–13 years.

In a very elegant experimental manipulation, either guppies or predators were moved from one natural setting to the other, and the breeding behavior of the guppies was observed over the ensuing years. As can be seen in the table, when guppies were moved from the lower pools, where adults are preyed upon, to the upper pools, after five years (approximately 20 guppy generations) the average breeding ages of both males and females had moved toward those characteristic of the upper pools. In an even more convincing demonstration, the predator *C. alta* was moved from the lower pools to the upper pools, where it immediately began to prey on adult guppies. (Presumably *R. harti* continued to prey on the young in these pools.) After eleven years of exposure to *C. alta*, the average ages for both males and females in the upper pools were indistinguishable from ages in the lower pools.

The results obtained by Reznick and his colleagues addressed the interaction of the timing of onset of reproductive activity with the timing and rate of death from accidental causes such as predation. They did not address the impact of these manipulations on maximal lifespan. Nevertheless, these results are entirely consistent with the predictions of various theories of the evolution of senescence (but of course do not necessarily prove them; experiments can only disprove theories, never prove them correct). In these experiments, given the number of generations involved in the natural selection process (especially over 11 years), it is entirely possible that new genetic variants were being produced and selected for, although as in the Drosophila experiments it is certainly also the case that existing variants already in the gene pool provided a major source of material for selection.

What might the nature of these various genes be? That is the question posed by those pursuing the nature of senescence and death at the level of molecular biology and genetics. It is one of the most intriguing pursuits in all of modern biology, taking researchers into areas that may seem at first to have nothing at all to do with questions about the end of life. One of the greatest surprises is that some of the answers to these questions may be found at the opposite end of life—at its very beginnings. We will explore this fascinating aspect of senescence in the next chapter.

Conclusions

Biologically, we are all composed of two quite separate and distinct compartments: the somatic and the germline. The only function of somatic cells is to act as guardians of the germline DNA; the somatic individual as such is little more than a somewhat fancy—and disposable—vehicle for that DNA. It is entirely in the interest of the genes being passed forward in the germ cells that the DNA in the somatic cells be destroyed. The somatic cells—the somatic *individuals*—of each generation become genetically irrelevant once those individuals' germ-cell DNA is recombined through sex with the DNA of others. Just as the macronuclei of paramecia are destroyed at the end of each generation, so too are somatic individuals. As sentient beings we may have come to regard our somatic selves—the part of us that thinks and reads, feels and loves—as the most important part of who we are. That is not nature's view.

The ability to isolate and compare genes from different animals has led to the creation of a new field of evolutionary studies called "molecular evolution." Over time, a gene arising in a common ancestor will gradually accumulate mutations as it descends through the various species arising from that ancestor. Since mutations arise at a more or less steady rate, the degree of molecular divergence of the same gene in different species is an approximate measure of the degree of evolutionary divergence and hence relatedness of those species. Not all genes evolve at the same rate, however. Some genes will have diverged considerably over time; the corresponding proteins appear to have a great deal of structural latitude, such that changes in structure do not necessarily compromise function. Other genes have much greater restrictions placed on them. A few genes have changed hardly at all over several billion years of evolution. We infer in such cases that the protein encoded by these genes must have worked well from the very beginning, and any changes in structure would have dire consequences for function. The study of genes and proteins has proved to be a valuable adjunct to classical evolutionary studies based on comparative anatomy and fossil relationships.

The molecular approach can also be used to gain valuable insights into biological processes such as aging. As we will see, the genes underlying senescence are already in place in the earliest eukaryotic organisms such as paramecia and yeast. Although numerous mutational changes have accumulated in these genes over evolutionary time, they are in fact remarkably conserved in species as diverse as worms and human beings. This consistency in the genes involved in senescence pathways among widely divergent organisms makes it difficult to imagine that random accretion of different senescence genes in various species across evolutionary time could have played a major role in the development of senescence as we find it today. If that were the case, we would expect the genes underlying senescence to be different in evolutionarily widely separated species. They are not. Addition of genes causing senescence through random accumulation—the gene for Huntington's disease is most often cited—may well have made a minor contribution to overall senescence. But a study of senescence at the molecular level is rapidly changing the way we think about the evolution of senescence. The data underlying this shift in evolutionary paradigm is presented in the following chapters.

4

Of Embryos and Worms and Very Old Men

The Developmental Genetics of Senescence and Lifespan

A major question that troubles those who think deeply about the evolutionary origins of senescence and death is the biological basis for the tremendous variability in maximum lifespan seen between species living in the same environmental niche. Why do some species live so much longer than others? How could such differences have arisen in the first place? Maximum lifespan will certainly be affected to some extent by variability in the rate at which senescence results in death, either through accident or collapse of internal systems, once it sets in. But perhaps more important, variability in maximum lifespan seems to reflect the variability in the time after birth before individual members of a given species reach reproductive maturity. Evidence gathered across a wide range of species suggests that truly "serious" senescence is delayed until at least the beginning of the reproductive period. To understand this latter point fully, let us explore for a moment not the development of senescence in different species through the course of evolutionary time (the *phylogeny* of senescence) but rather the history of senescence within the developmental framework of a single individual—the *ontogeny* of senescence.

Although entirely mortal, we ourselves arise from cells that are potentially immortal: not, as is commonly assumed, the haploid germ cells (sperm or ova) of our parents, but rather the cells arising from the first few rounds of cell division after those germ cells unite in fertilization to form a diploid, single-cell zygote. The DNA passed to the next generation through the germ cells achieves its own biochemical immortality, but the germ cells themselves are, as cells, clearly only immortal in a philosophical sense. If removed from the body and grown in culture dishes, they have no more potential for unlimited cell growth than somatic cells.

Yet mature germ cells are in a sense poised on the edge of cellular immortality: Their immediate descendents, arising from the first post-fertilization divisions of the diploid zygote, can be isolated and placed into tissue culture, where they display the ability to replicate indefinitely. As long as care is taken to prevent them from following their natural tendency to press forward and form an embryo, they will continue to divide, as far as we can tell, without ever undergoing senescence. But when these zygote-derived cells complete their transition into *us*, some nine months later, none of our cells, including our germ cells, retain this kind of immortality. Descendents of our own *potentially* immortal germ cells can once again achieve transient cellular immortality, but only through fusion with the germ cells of another individual. The rest of us—our somatic selves—will age and die. How does this come about? What did we (the somatic we) lose—or gain—in those first few hours of uterine existence that will one day cost us our mortal lives?

An analysis of senescence through a study of these very early stages of animal development may turn out to be one of the most promising approaches to understanding how we age as adults. The laboratory subject of these analyses is something called embryonal stem (ES) cells. ES cells represent a stage of post-fertilization development that occurs in all mammals (and probably all vertebrates), but that has been studied most intensely in the mouse. ES cells are obtained by removing the early, rapidly dividing cell mass arising from the zygote (the blastula) as it moves down the Fallopian tubes toward the uterus, where it would normally implant and develop into a true embryo.

If these preimplantation cells are harvested during transit, and dispersed and placed in culture under appropriate conditions, they will continue to divide. The progeny of each cell will try hard to form a three-dimensional, self-adhering cell mass, or colony, which in turn strives mightily to turn itself into an embryo. The cells cannot do this in vitro, but they try. By continually collecting the colonies while they are small, redispersing the cells, and adjusting the culture medium in a way that disfavors the initiation of embryonic development, the cells can be held in an undifferentiated state indefinitely.

The value of ES cells as an experimental tool was initially recognized as a way to produce genetically altered mice. It has been possible to "knock out" specific genes from the DNA of ES cells grown in the laboratory, and then to reintroduce the genetically altered cells into a normally developing embryo, where they participate in formation of the various embryonic tissues and organs (Fig. 4.1). This is done by harvesting intact blastulas from a second, recently impregnated mouse that are at the same stage (approximately 100 cells) as the blastula from which the ES cells were originally obtained. The altered ES cells are carefully injected into this blastula, and the resulting genetically mosaic blastula is reimplanted into a foster mother. From a developmental point of view, no distinction is made between the host blastula and donor ES cells. When her babies are born, they, like the blastula they are derived from, will be mosaic; some of the cells in their bodies will

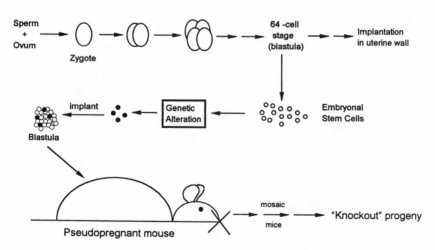

Figure 4.1. Embryonal stem cells. See text for details.

have descended from the altered ES cells, and some from the cells of the blastula into which the ES cells were injected. Of particular interest, some of the mosaic babies will, by chance, have germ cells derived from the altered ES cells; by mating such mice it is possible eventually to derive a line of mice in which all cells in the body lack the gene that has been knocked out. Such "knockout mice" have proved to be an extraordinarily useful tool for determining the function of a number of important genes, including those involved in senescence.

But our understanding of what ES cells are, and how they work, raises quite separate and very interesting questions about the origin and nature of senescence, and at the same time offers an ideal system in which to search for the answers. It is generally agreed that the germ cells prior to fertilization were not immortal (in a cellular sense); that zygote-derived cells at the ES-cell stage are immortal (or at least not subject to replicative senescence); and that this immortality is lost in subsequent embryonic development. It is of great interest to cell biologists that ES cells seem to represent a state of truly inherent immortality. Cancer cells and certain virally infected (virally transformed) cells also exhibit replicative immortality, but this state must be induced either by mutation (cancer), or through the action of virally borne genes. The immortality of ES cells is an entirely natural state of the cell at that stage of its development. There are now established lines of mouse ES cells that have been in more or less continuously replicating culture for ten years or more, with no signs of senescence, while retaining full potential to give rise to a complete and functioning mouse.

We do not know precisely where during embryonic development immortality is lost, although there is good reason to believe it is quite early, probably at about the time the growing embryonal cell mass implants in the uterine wall. Embryonic development proceeds by a process referred to as differentiation. Cells at the ES cell stage are undifferentiated and totipotent; that is, any one of them has the potential to develop into any cell or tissue characteristic of the adult body. However, as embryonic development proceeds, through cell division and differentiation, each embryonic cell gradually gives up some of its "potency" on its way to becoming a particular type of end-stage cell: a liver cell, say, or a kidney or blood cell.

The gradual restriction of developmental potential through time at the cellular level reflects events occurring in the DNA within each of the developing cells. One of the things that happens during embryonic development and differentiation is a gradual shutting down of portions of the genome. Embryonic cells at or before the stage represented by ES cells appear to have what we might call a fully "open genome": essentially all of the genes of the genome are open and accessible, able to contribute equally to the various structural and functional components of the new individual. This does not mean that all of the genes are actively expressed, but simply that they could be, with relatively little effort by the cell.

Many genes in the genome—the majority, in fact—are involved with the basic structure and operation of any cell type, and are expressed in all cells throughout the body; these are the so-called housekeeping genes. These genes remain in the open state throughout the life of the cell. There is a second category of genes, however, which we can call special-function genes. These are the genes that dictate the unique characteristics of the various tissues of the body; lung, brain, heart, and so forth. While carried in all cells of the body (because all cells of the body carry the entire genome in their nuclei), during embryonic development the vast majority of these special-function genes become increasingly inaccessible in different emerging cell lines, until the cells of a given tissue or organ express only the specific function genes for that tissue or organ. All cells of the body, for example, have the gene for insulin present in their DNA. Only the ß cells of the endocrine pancreas, however, maintain this gene in an open, readable form at all times.

Understanding the difference between housekeeping and special-function genes is crucial to the cellular and molecular approach to understanding senescence. When we add up all of the outward manifestations of aging, and combine them with all of the internal age-related changes detectable by laboratory tests, we end up with a staggeringly long list of changes associated with the aging process. It has seemed to some gerontologists that an enormous number of different processes must be taking place during aging in the various tissues and cells of the body to explain such a diversity of measurable events. Yet this need not necessarily be the case. The vast majority of genes expressed in any given cell will be the housekeeping genes, and at this level gene expression in the different cells of the body actually differs by very little. All cells, by definition, express the same housekeeping genes. It is only a relative handful of specialty genes that make our various cells—liver versus lung, brain versus muscle—different from one another. In each cell, the housekeeping genes support and sustain the functions of the specialty genes.

It is the nature of housekeeping genes that allows us to understand how a defect in even a single gene could have widespread and varied effects on aging phenotypes. For example, imagine a housekeeping gene, "X," whose function is to regulate energy production in each cell of the body. In the absence of energy, cells are simply unable to carry out their assigned function, whatever that function may be. So if the ability of our gene X to function is somehow decreased in all cells with age, then the ability of those cells to do their job will also decrease with age. Skin cells may produce less collagen; hair cells may not be able to produce coloring pigment; muscle cells or brain cells may no longer operate at maximal levels. In every cell, there is but a single gene defect, and it is the same defect in every cell. The result in terms of aging phenotypes will seem to be very different in each of these cells, yet each of these phenotypes resulted from the altered activity of a single gene.

But let us return to the developing embryo. Embryonic cells travel along different developmental pathways, but they all proceed from totipotency to pluripotency (having a relatively limited potential for further development), and eventually become monopotent: highly differentiated, specific cell types with specialty gene expression limited to those carrying out the special functions of that particular cell, and no potential for further or alternate cellular development. A kidney cell, once fully differentiated, no longer has the capacity to become a lung cell; a brain cell can never become a blood cell. All of the genes that were originally present in the open genome—including all of the specialty genes—are still physically present in every fully differentiated cell, but in each such cell the vast majority of the specialty genes are in a greatly repressed and inaccessible state. Only those specialty genes directly related to a cell's fully differentiated functions are actively expressed.

Somewhere near the beginning of this transition from totipotency to the final differentiated state, the replicatively immortal cells derived from the zygote become mortal. It may very well be that it is here, at the very beginning of life, that the process of senescence actually begins. Understanding how this takes place is one of the most active areas of contemporary biological research. The hypothesis most consistent with the facts we have in hand, which we will examine in the remainder of this book, is that the program for senescence is actually present and operational even in the apparently immortal early embryo cells, but that this program is effectively neutralized by what we can think of as senescence repressor genes—genes whose products interfere with expression of the senescence program. Under this scenario, there would be sets of genes—we can call them senescence effector genes—whose expression initiates senescence and sets the stage for the ultimate death of the cell.

Aging at the cellular level is seen as a balancing act between these two sets of genes. In fully open genomes, like those found in the earliest embryonic cells, the senescence repressor genes function at full force, completely blocking senescence; as long as these genes are expressed, the cells are effectively immortal because the senescence program cannot be initiated (Fig. 4.2). As the cells begin to differentiate, and turn off various unused special function genes, the senescence repressor genes are presumed to be "turned down" considerably, but not fully; although senescence probably operates to some extent in the

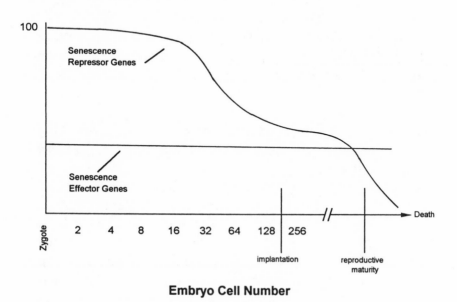

Figure 4.2. Changes in senescence-related genes during the life history of an animal.

embryo and on up through the pre-reproductive years, it is expressed in full force only once reproductive maturity has been achieved. The senescence effector genes themselves, under this scenario, are never actually shut off; their effect prior to the start of differentiation, and in the pre-reproductive years, is simply blocked or at least modulated by senescence repressor genes. We will explore the precise nature of genes that trigger and repress senescence later in this chapter, and throughout the book.

This increased understanding of the gain and loss of immortality during embryonic development provides a possible basis for understanding, at a mechanistic level, the relationship of senescence and lifespan in the adult. One biological basis for the differences in lifespan among different species could be differences in the delay in turning off, or turning off fully, the senescence-repressing genes expressed in all cells shortly after conception. The delay would be related to the time needed for the individual to reach reproductive maturity, and begin the process of generating at least a replacement level of offspring. The overall expression of senescence throughout the life history of an organism would reflect an interaction of three classes of senescence genes. The senescence effector genes are responsible for triggering the cellular damage leading to the senescent state. Their expression begins at conception, but their effect is completely repressed, at least transiently, by senescence repressor genes. Probably at about the time of uterine implantation, the senescence repressor genes ease back somewhat, and a low level of senescence begins to be expressed. Finally, at about the time of sexual maturity, a third class of genes, senescence regulatory genes, comes into play. These genes either turn off the senescence repressor genes or greatly attenuate their activity, allowing senescence to begin operating in earnest. The timing of the onset of the effect of this third set of genes is closely related to sexual maturation, and these regulatory genes—at least in mammals—may be identical with the genes that control expression of reproductive hormones. This aspect of lifespan—essentially, the distance between the two vertical bars along the age axis in Fig. 4.2—is under strict genetic control, and ultimately accounts for the differences we see in maximal lifespan.

But why would such widely varying delays occur? What could be the value of a prolonged pre-reproductive phase? From an evolutionary point of view, there is no inherent advantage in delaying the time of transmission of DNA from one generation to the next. Once new genetic possibilities have been created, either by random mutation or by sexual recombination, they must be tested against the environment. Mutations that would increase the pre-reproductive lifespan of the individual housing these new possibilities are of no inherent value, *unless* they in some way increase the efficiency with which the inherited DNA will be passed on to yet another generation. At one level, extremely rapid reproduction, of the type seen in the very simplest living organisms, has a strong advantage in that the DNA those organisms are responsible for transmitting has more opportunities over a given period of time to try new rearrangements of itself. In the competition for securing an ecological niche this may impart definite advantages. What kinds of advantages could be conferred by a longer pre-reproductive period that would outweigh the advantages of rapid reproduction? Given that natural selection can act only on genetic changes affecting reproductive efficiency, how could a longer pre-reproductive period increase that efficiency?

We do not know. There are a number of characteristics that correlate with increased maximum lifespan, but it is easy to confuse cause with effect, and we often do not know which is which. For example, one feature of organisms that have larger maximum lifespan values is that they produce many fewer offspring per individual than do organisms with shorter lifespans. They have somehow increased the efficiency of the reproductive process. The advantage of increased efficiency is that fewer resources are required to maintain a stable or increasing population level. Implicit in this is that the offspring are much less likely to die by accidental means prior to their own reproductive maturity, and in fact increased maximum lifespan occurs only in populations with lower levels of predation and other causes of accidental death. Whereas a pair of mice may have to produce forty copies of themselves to maintain a steady population level, a pair of humans may have to produce only three. Across a wide range of species, there is a correlation of maximum lifespan with reproductive efficiency and low accidental death rates. But why should increased reproductive efficiency per se delay the onset of reproduction itself, and thus of senescence? What cellular or molecular mechanisms can we imagine would underlie such a cause-and-effect relationship?

There is also a correlation of maximum lifespan with the length of time individuals actually spend in producing offspring, and rearing them to independence. Reproductively more efficient species tend to devote much more time to the bearing and rearing of fewer offspring. It has been argued that the additional time spent with each offspring allows time for parents to teach offspring how to cope more effectively with their environment. But why this would be any more advantageous in the transmission of DNA than simply producing large numbers of offspring and setting them free to compete for survival is not at all clear. And again, how could we explain this at a mechanistic level? Correlations of various parameters related to the evolution of reproductive patterns, senescence, and lifespan are important in setting the overall framework for the way a given system actually works, but, like the theories of the evolution of senescence discussed earlier, they provide little insight into the mechanisms that may have brought it all about.

What is clear in eukaryotic cells and organisms is that *death is the default state*. If we do not die from accidental causes, our cells—and we—will one day die from the cumulative effects of senescence; what is politely called "natural death" or simply "old age." From the moment the transient immortal state of the immediate descendents of the germ cells is ended, all eukaryotic cells begin to die; it is simply a matter of time. In some species, individuals are ready to reproduce within hours of birth; in other species, reproductive maturity may require years. Until that point, the senescence repressor genes, which maintain a state of effective immortality in early embryos, greatly retard expression of the senescence program in young adults. Each species has worked out a program of juggling the initiation and repression of senescence that is optimum for its survival, and for transmission of its DNA to the next generation. Such programs may or may not include a long lifespan.

As the Worm Turns: Genetic Control of Senescence and Lifespan in Caenorhabditis elegans

It is all well and good to talk about senescence effector and repressor genes, but what exactly might the nature of such genes be? Do they really exist, and, if so, what do they do and how do they fit into the overall biology of living cells? Are they dedicated exclusively to aging, or might they play other roles as well?

68

In the past decade or so, we have learned a great deal about the genes involved in senescence. Somewhat surprisingly, we see almost exactly the same genes at work in an amazingly wide range of different organisms. Aging and death in eukaryotic organisms seems to be very important in nature, and the genes responsible for particularly critical functions are generally highly conserved in evolution. For example, the genes responsible for replicative senescence in paramecia and yeast have been highly conserved throughout all of eukaryotic evolution, and the very same genes—in slightly modified but definitely recognizable form—can be seen in humans today. These genes in unicellular organisms are essentially death genes; in a single cell, death of a cell is equivalent to death of the organism. But what about multicellular organisms that arose from single-cell eukaryotic ancestors? Some of our most sophisticated information about the genetic regulation of lifespan and death in higher animals comes from studying one of the lowliest of multicellular eukaryotic organisms: the nematode worm *Caenorhabditis elegans.*

C. elegans is one of the most intensely studied of the primitive multicellular eukaryotes. Its value as a model system for many different aspects of eukaryotic biology was made evident in a powerful way by the British scientist Sydney Brenner. Brenner had been trained in the emerging field of molecular biology just as it reached its apotheosis with the unraveling of the structure and function of DNA and the deciphering of the genetic code. Others would continue to unravel in ever finer detail exactly how genes work at a mechanistic level, but Brenner was looking far beyond the chemistry of genes; he was interested in how genes could guide the development of a complex multicellular organism. Until Brenner's time, scientists had worked almost exclusively in bacteria and yeast, for one simple reason: They could dissect these organisms through their genetics. But Brenner saw that the challenges of the future would lie in unraveling the function of more complex eukaryotes. Brenner wanted to know, for example, how genes could specify the structure and function of something as complex as the nervous system. To do this he wanted to work with a model eukaryote in which he could apply the genetics that had worked so well in prokaryotes.

Genetics requires the transmission and segregation of traits over many consecutive generations, so Brenner wanted an organism with both a nervous system and a short generation time. *C. elegans* seemed ideal. It is extremely small (1.2 mm in length), the entire organism consisting of less than 1000 cells. It reaches sexual maturity in just over three days, with an average life span of about thirteen days. It grows in the soil in the wild, and is easy to maintain in the laboratory, feeding on common bacteria such as *Escherichia coli*. It is a self-fertilizing hermaphrodite with occasionally occurring males, which makes genetic analysis much easier. It has six chromosomes, and an estimated 18,000 genes.

Brenner published his first detailed genetic dissection of *C. elegans* in 1974, and over the next several years its value as an experimental system was perceived by researchers in a number of different fields. Most important, developmental biologists studied the generation of adult organisms from the initial egg, and have traced the origin and fate of every single cell throughout the *C. elegans* lifespan. This is the only multicellular eukaryote for which such extensive "fate mapping" of a developing organism has been carried out. The adult worm contains exactly 959 cells, of which 302 cells comprise the nervous system. But during the development of the adult, an additional 131 cells are generated that never show up in the adult worm. Like the cells that form the webbing between the fingers of a human hand, these cells commit suicide, dying of apoptosis over a six- to eight-hour period. However, in the adult, none of the cells that survive are dividing. This is important, because it gives scientists a chance to look at the senescence process in nondividing cells.

The genes involved in initiating and resisting cell death in *C. elegans* have been analyzed in detail over the past ten years, primarily in the laboratory of Robert Horwitz at the Massachusetts Institute of Technology. By studying mutant worms in which the 131 condemned cells failed to die according to plan, Horvitz and his students discovered a number of key genes that control the death program. Two genes, called ced-3 and ced-4, were identified as causative in the programmed cell death that occurs during embryonic development. If either gene is mutant, the cells fail to die, and proceed to develop into superfluous cells for which the worm has no use. Certainly in terms of the life history of individual cells, these genes qualify as senescence effector genes. In the course of their studies, the researchers discovered another gene, called ced-9, that opposes the action of ced-3 and -4 in cells, and would thus qualify as a senescence-repressor gene.

The incredible evolutionary conservatism of such genes is revealed by the fact that the human homologue of the ced-9 gene, called bcl-2, can be transferred into *C. elegans* worms lacking ced-9, where it is able to block the actions of the worm's ced-3 and -4 gene products! Humans also have molecular analogs of the ced-3 gene that actively promote apoptosis in cells instructed to commit suicide. The *C. elegans* genes also work in mammalian cells. Given that humans and *C. elegans* are separated by nearly a billion years of evolution, it is incredible that the genes for cell death can be exchanged so easily between them. Perhaps this is telling us just how important cell death has been throughout the history of multicellular animals.

Exactly what these genes and their products do inside cells that leads to cell death is one of the most active areas of biological research, and is currently being worked out in laboratories around the world. It seems very likely that they function in or near cellular organelles called mitochondria, which are involved in energy production within the cell. Among the by-products of energy production are a number of highly corrosive forms of oxygen that are thought to promote cellular aging through oxidative damage to DNA and other cellular molecules. One possibility for the function of these genes is that they modulate this damage, which can rapidly become lethal for a cell.

C. elegans has also provided us with one of our first looks at genes that control senescence and lifespan of the whole organism, including its nondividing cells. One such gene, called age-1, was first described by researchers in 1988. Certain mutations in age-1 result in a doubling of the maximum lifespan for *C. elegans*, from twenty-two to forty-six days; the observed increase in lifespan occurs almost entirely in the post-reproductive stages of the life cycle. The fact that the mutated gene results in an increased maximum lifespan suggests the function of the normal gene may be to inhibit the function of senescence repressor genes in *C. elegans*. A close study of this gene suggests that it, too, regulates the cell's ability to deal with the toxic oxygen by-products of energy metabolism.

The age-1 mutation was readily produced in the laboratory, and it is difficult to imagine that it would not on occasion arise spontaneously in nature. The extended lifespan caused by this mutation would seem at one level to be advantageous for the individual; yet this mutation appears not to have been positively selected in evolution. This is a strong argument that a prolonged lifespan for individuals is not perceived by nature as a priori advantageous, and may actually be selected *against*, by limiting the production within cells of substances that could increase maximum lifespan unnecessarily.

In addition to age-1, there is a series of genes in *C. elegans* referred to collectively as "clock" genes. These genes seem to function by somehow regulating the rate of progress through the various stages of the *C. elegans* life cycle. Appropriate combinations of alleles of the clock genes can increase average and maximal lifespan up to four-fold. One of these genes, called clk-1, was recently cloned and examined in some detail. The same gene was found to occur in a wide range of species, including yeast, mice, and humans, and is highly conserved. Little is known directly about these genes in humans, but the mouse and yeast genes resembling clk-1 appear to be involved in controlling the pace of metabolism within a cell. This would be consistent with what has been observed in *C. elegans* itself, where clk-1 controls the pace at which the worms proceed through each of their distinct life phases.

Whether the equivalent of the clk-1 gene plays a similar role in higher animals, perhaps including humans, is currently the subject of intense investigation. The possibility of specific genes that could control the pace of aging in humans is obviously of great interest, and we begin our investigation of this question in the next chapter.

5

Human Genetic Diseases That Mimic the Aging Process

The search for genes that might be involved in the human aging process—human senescence—was given a major push forward with the publication, in 1978, of a landmark study by George Martin entitled "Genetic Syndromes in Man with Potential Relevance to the Pathobiology of Aging." His analysis of the existing medical and scientific literature had suggested that as many as 7000 human genes might be involved in the degenerative processes associated with aging, but he concluded that probably no more than seventy, and perhaps as few as seven, of these genes controlled processes in the body that have a major impact on senescence. He excluded from consideration genes encoding specific diseases that might cause death either early or late in life; although death is clearly the endpoint of senescence, Martin was more interested in the *process* of senescence, as defined by studies in both animals and humans.*

---

*This may be too narrow a view of senescence. As discussed earlier, internally pro-

One of the major conclusions Martin was able to reach as a result of his analysis was that although aging-like symptoms can be found in a number of different genetic diseases, no single disease can be said to mimic completely all of the known parameters of the human aging process. There is no single "aging gene" that determines human life-span and regulates human senescence. Nevertheless, Martin identified ten well-known genetic diseases in which there was an accelerated progression of a large number of distinct aging traits (Table 5.1). Because each of these diseases involves only certain aspects of the aging process, he called them segmental progerias; progeria is a Greek term meaning "early aging." Seven of these disorders are known or presumed single-gene defects; three are chromosomal aneuploidies, meaning there are extra, missing, or malformed chromosomes.

In addition to helping focus the search for genes that might underlie the human aging process, Martin's analysis also raised some interesting questions about the nature of the aging process itself. For instance, if many of the various symptoms accompanying each of the disorders listed in Table 5.1 reflect a normal part of the aging process, why are they referred to as diseases? Should aging be regarded as a disease? Martin himself, like many others who study senescence, referred repeatedly to the "pathobiology" of aging—it is even in the title of his paper. Another question raised by the focus on genes associated with senescence is how relevant such genetic diseases could be to normal human aging. The diseases in Table 5.1 presumably involve genes that are mutated; does normal human aging involve mutated genes? Are these (and perhaps other) genes organized into some sort of "program" that, in the totality of its execution, leads to human senescence and death?

Before attempting to answer these questions, it will be useful to have a closer look at some of the diseases identified by Martin as mimicking the human aging process. To place the description of these diseases in some sort of perspective, we will begin with a very brief discussion of the nature of disease itself.

---

grammed events in an organism that lead to a lethal idiopathic disease, or increase susceptibility to death through external disease or accident, should probably be considered part of the overall senescence program of that organism.

Table 5.1. *Human genetic disorders reflecting various aspects of the human aging process*[a]

Known single-gene defects	Principle senescence-related features
Ataxia telangectasia	Senile dementia; diabetes
Myotonic dystrophy	Diabetes; hair graying; cataracts
Werner syndrome	Wrinkled skin; hair graying and loss; atherosclerosis; cataracts; cancer; diabetes; osteoporosis
Presumed single-gene defects	
Hutchinson-Gilford syndrome	Wrinkled skin; hair loss; atherosclerosis; osteoporosis; hypertension
Cockayne syndrome	Senile dementia; U.V. sensitivity; cataracts; osteoporosis; hypertension
Seip syndrome	Hypertension; diabetes; dementia
Familial cervical lipodysplasia	Diabetes; arthritis; hair loss; dementia
Chromosomal aneuploidies	
Down syndrome	Senile dementia; cataracts; diabetes; hair graying; cancer
Klinefelter syndrome	Diabetes; hair graying; cancer
Turner syndrome	Hypertension; diabetes; cancer

[a]Disorders are listed as known single-gene defects where the causative gene has been isolated and identified. The presumption of a single-gene defect is based on genetic mapping studies. Of the aneuploidies with progeric features, Down syndrome individuals have an extra chromosome 21 ("trisomy 21"). Individuals with Klinefelter syndrome are males with 1–3 additional X chromosomes. In Turner syndrome, females have only one X chromosome ("X0"). Diabetes, where indicated, is type II, or maturity onset. Senile dementia may include any of a number of changes in brain tissue associated with dementia.

Although enormous in both number and complexity, all human diseases derive from two fundamentally different sources. Either they are caused by external agents or they arise through some inherent defect in the human organism itself. External agents include such things as deprivation of food or water; extremes of temperature or radiation; chemicals in the environment, whether natural or man-made, that disturb the body's own internal chemistry; and infectious microorganisms. The latter group encompasses a wide range of bacteria, viruses, funguses, and parasites that find the warm, well-regulated, food-rich mammalian body a perfect place to live and reproduce. Some of these "microbes" have learned to live in harmony with their hosts, causing no harm; a few even play a positive role, such as helping to digest food. But a great many others can cause considerable harm, in the form of what we call infectious disease. Prior to the early part of the twentieth century and the advent of effective public health and vaccination programs, infectious disease was a major source of morbidity and mortality in humans.

But when all of the diseases caused by external agents are added up, a very large number of human maladies remain unaccounted for. These *idiopathic diseases* were once written off as being of unknown origin, but most of them are now thought to be due to alterations in the genes that encode all of the proteins needed to construct and operate a living organism. Virtually unknown a hundred years ago, today we understand that genes are specific chemical sequences written in the language of DNA, and carried in every cell of the body. Human beings have on the order of 100,000 genes contained in twenty-three pairs of structures called chromosomes. The DNA sequences defining these genes are passed from generation to generation during reproduction, and account for the similarities (and differences) between parent and offspring. However, over time these sequences can change. Changes may arise in DNA accidentally, through mutation, or purposely, as part of the reproductive process. The generation of genetic changes that can be acted on by natural selection is a vital part of the process of evolution, allowing organisms to adapt over time to changes in their environment.

With evolutionary time, a given species will have tried and discarded many different forms (alleles) of its component genes in an attempt to secure its place within a given environmental niche. These genetic changes, whether occurring by accident or through purposeful reproductive means, are an ongoing process. If harmful genetic mutations occur in a gene housed in any of the cells of the body other than a sperm or an ovum, i.e., in a somatic cell), the results could well be lethal, but only for the cell in which it occurs or any of its immediate descendants. Since most somatic cells in an adult organism divide rarely or not at all, the number of cells affected by somatic mutations is usually quite limited.* Such mutations are rarely even detectable. But when mutations occur in germ cells, they are passed on to all of the offspring of the individual in whom the mutation occurred. And because those offspring derive entirely from the DNA inherited through the germ cells, every single cell in their bodies will have the mutated form of the gene in question. Including, it should be pointed out, their own germ cells: this is the origin of what we call inherited genetic diseases, human disorders that are passed forward from generation to generation.

There is one additional point in the life cycle of an individual when mutations may arise, and it is an important one. If a harmful mutational event occurs during fetal development, even if it occurs in only a single somatic cell, a significant proportion of the cells of the resulting individual may be affected. At the fetal stage, most of the cells of the growing body are vigorously dividing and, particularly early in development, each dividing cell may have a great many descendents. If the mutation is not developmentally lethal, as in the case of a gene that is not expressed until later in life, the embryo will not abort. But the earlier in embryological life such a mutation occurs, the more cells will be involved. This type of mutation can give rise to what are sometimes referred to as sporadic genetic diseases; diseases caused by defective genes that affect major portions of the body—including entire organs—but which are not inherited. Certain occurences of Alzheimer's disease may reflect a sporadic mutational event.

There are an estimated 4000 inherited genetic diseases in the human species. Some of these, like cystic fibrosis, sickle-cell anemia, or Tay-Sach's disease, are caused by defects in a single gene. Other such diseases, like diabetes, involve multiple defective genes. These genetic defects may be either dominant or recessive; this distinction is important, so let us take a moment to define it clearly. Like virtually all other eukaryotes, humans are diploid; we have two copies of each gene stored in the DNA in each cell. If one of them becomes defective (is mutated

---

*A major exception is cells of the blood system and the immune system, many of which divide throughout life. Here somatic mutations occur continuously, and in fact are an important mechanism of diversification in the immune system. For further information, see William R. Clark, *At War Within: The Double-Edged Sword of Immunity* (New York: Oxford University Press, 1995).

in such a way that the protein it produces doesn't function properly), in most cases this is simply not noticed; the other copy of the same gene can make enough normal copies of the protein to keep the cell running. It is only when both copies of the gene are mutated that a problem arises, because then there are no normal copies of the protein available to the cell. Such mutations are called recessive. Diseases caused by recessive mutations are rare, because the likelihood of both gene copies being damaged is extremely small.

On the other hand, occasionally an altered protein produced by a mutant gene will, either directly or indirectly, interfere with the function of the normal protein made by the other gene; only one gene copy is dysfunctional, but the cellular function encoded by that gene is shut down even though the other gene copy is perfectly normal. These kinds of mutations are called dominant (or sometimes "dominant-negative"). To inherit a recessive genetic disease (cystic fibrosis, for example), it is necessary to inherit a "bad" gene copy from each parent. In a dominant genetic disease (like Huntington's disease), the inheritance of a single bad gene copy from either parent is sufficient to cause the disease.

There is one other parameter of inherited genetic diseases that should be defined: They may be either autosomal or sex-linked. Human genes are arrayed along twenty-three pairs of chromosomes. In twenty-two of these pairs, the chromosomes are identical. The twenty-third "pair" is not really a pair; these are the so-called "X" and "Y" chromosomes that determine an individual's gender. Someone who inherits two X chromosomes is "X-X" and female; someone who is "X-Y" is male. If a gene residing on the X chromosome undergoes a recessive mutation, a female "carrier" of this mutation does not have a problem, because she has two X chromosomes. However, a male carrying the same chromosome will experience the underlying disease, since he will not have a compensating additional X chromosome. The mutation in effect becomes dominant. Mutations of genes lying on the X or Y chromosomes may thus lead to sex-linked genetic diseases like hemophilia A or Duchenne muscular dystrophy; alterations in genes on any of the other twenty-two pairs of autosomal chromosomes may give rise to autosomal genetic diseases. Recessive genetic diseases are almost always autosomal.

Whatever the origin of a defective gene, disease arises when the protein encoded by that gene, needed to carry out a critical function in the body, is not available. If the protein is crucial during fetal development, its loss may give rise to what is called a developmental lethal, in which case it does not cause a disease per se; the fetus simply aborts and the underlying cause is rarely perceived. If the fetus survives in the womb, it may be born and manifest symptoms of the disease essentially from birth, or disease symptoms may appear only later in life.

As we saw in the previous chapter, everything we know about human senescence, and about the determination of lifespan in general, suggests that it is internally regulated, which means that ultimately it must reflect events at the level of genes and DNA. How are instructions for the aging process written into our genes? What might such a program look like? How would it operate, and how is it regulated through time? The segmental progerias presented in Table 5.1 are thought by many to represent various portions of an aging program in humans. Before we discuss the merits of this hypothesis, let's continue with a closer examination of just what is involved in a few of these diseases.

The Hutchinson–Gilford Progeria Syndrome

The first formal description of what would come to be known as a progeric syndrome was presented at a meeting of the Royal Medical and Chirurgical Society in 1886 by the renowned English physician-surgeon Jonathon Hutchinson. Born in 1828 into a Quaker family in Yorkshire, Hutchinson received his formal medical training at the prestigious St. Bartholomew's Hospital in London. He was subsequently appointed a Professor of Surgery at London Hospital, but his interests ranged over the entire field of medical inquiry. Although elected a Fellow (and later President) of the Royal College of Surgeons, his most important contributions were in the study of venereal disease, especially congenital syphilis. But he published over 1000 papers before his death in 1913 in areas as disparate as ophthalmology and dermatology, surgery and neurology. It is perhaps no wonder, then, that his far-roving eye would be the first to detect a case of progeria, described in "Congenital Absence of Hair, with Atrophied Condition of the Skin and Its Appendages." In his presentation to his medical colleagues in 1886, Hutchinson described "the case of a boy three and a half years old, who presented a very withered 'old-mannish' appearance. His skin was remarkably thin, in some places not being thicker than brown paper. The genitals presented a marked contrast to the rest of the body, being in a state of a normally plump child. He had no nipples, their sites being occupied by little patches of scar."

This report lay largely unremarked upon in the medical literature until, in 1904, another English physician, Hastings Gilford, described a second case. This patient was also a male, although not seen by Gilford until he was fourteen years old. Gilford also examined Hutchinson's patient, who was by then fifteen years of age. Hutchinson's patient died at age seventeen; Gilford's at age eighteen. Like Hutchinson, Gilford noted the wizened appearance, the aged condition of the skin, growth retardation, and general lack of hair and body fat. But he also reported that at autopsy his patient had a normal (e.g., young-appearing) brain, liver, and genitalia. It was Gilford who first suggested the term progeria for this condition. Gilford wrote a lengthy and scholarly paper on these two patients, and tried to put their cases into the context of disorders of accelerated senescence. He commented that no cases had been reported prior to Hutchinson's 1886 paper, even in the popular literature on "medical curiosities"; nevertheless, Gilford felt the two patients were so similar that they could not represent random events, but must be suffering from the same disease.

The descriptions provided by Hutchinson and Gilford in their initial reports could be used to diagnose this form of progeria today, and the disorder they described is formally referred to as the Hutchinson-Gilford progeria syndrome (HGPS.) The addition of some seventy or so well-described cases since their initial reports does allow a slightly more detailed picture to be drawn, however. First, it is clear that this is an exceedingly rare disease; the frequency is estimated at perhaps one in a million live births in the United States. It is now apparent that males and females are affected equally, and there is no discernible racial correlation. Most HG progerics appear relatively normal at birth. The only signs of a possible problem during the first few months of life are a faint cyanosis (slight blue coloring) of the mid-facial region, and a failure of the skull bones to fuse together properly after birth. In fact, the two patients seen by Gilford at ages fourteen and fifteen still had small but detectable openings at the front of the skulltop.

Although the time of onset of more definitive symptoms varies from case to case (ranging from the day of birth to ten months or so of age), generally by the end of the first year there is noticeable growth retardation and the appearance of physical features commonly associated with HGPS (Fig. 5.1). HG progerics only rarely exceed four feet in height during their brief lives. All body hair, including the eyebrows and eyelashes, either fails to develop or is lost; any hair that remains on the head is white and usually described as "downy" or "fuzz-like." There are also skeletal and structural abnormalities. These may be relatively minor, such as the receding chin, large cranium, beak-like nose and protruding eyes seen in almost all HG progerics. These features are caused by the slow growth of facial bones, including the teeth, and wasting of facial flesh; the comparatively normal size of the rest of the skull results in what have been described as small, bird-like faces.

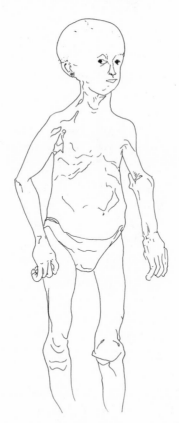

Figure 5.1. Thirteen-year-old male child with Hutchison-Gilford progeria. (Drawn by Celine Park)

Voices are usually thin and high-pitched. Other physical problems are more serious and debilitating: the long bones are lacking in proper calcification, and as a result are thinner and shorter than normal. The collar bones often fail to develop properly, causing the shoulder and chest areas to appear narrow. The fingers and toes are usually very short, due to degeneration and resorption of the distal bones. In most cases there is marked degeneration of the hip structure, resulting in a "bow-legged" condition. Elbow and knee joints are of normal size, but tend to fill with fibrotic scar tissue, giving them a swollen appearance and making limb movement difficult. Overall, the apparent physical similarity of HG progerics is rather startling; it is often said of them that they look more like one another than like other members of their own families.

Some of the most striking changes take place in the skin. The subcutaneous layers, with their fat and nutritive cells, degenerate; the remaining superficial layers of the skin become thin, rather dry, and somewhat transparent. (As noted by both Hutchinson and Gilford, these changes often do not extend to the pubic region.) Thus one of the characteristic features of progeric children, in addition to their baldness, is the visual prominence of numerous veins, particularly in the scalp. The skin itself becomes wrinkled and lacking in tone, exhibits "liver spot" discolorations, and heals poorly. These changes involve all regions of the body, and mimic quite closely changes in the skin normally seen in very old adults.

Children with HGPS have an average lifespan of twelve to thirteen years; survival beyond twenty years is rare. They never develop sexually. Voices do not deepen in males; females do not develop breasts; neither sex develops hair associated with sexual maturation. (The absence of nipples remarked by Hutchinson is seen in about half of affected individuals.) In cases examined at autopsy, the germ cells (sperm and ova) are also clearly incapable of reproductive function, and no individual with HGPS has ever produced children. They are of normal intelligence throughout life, and their personalities are also remarkably normal in light of their condition, of which they are entirely aware. HG progerics appear to proceed directly from childhood to old age, without ever passing through adolescence or young adulthood. It is for this reason that HGPS has been proposed to represent both a precocious (early onset) and accelerated manifestation of at least some portions of the normal human aging process. And indeed, nearly all progerics die at the end of their brief lives of the same causes as the truly aged: most from heart attacks or strokes, a few from congestive heart failure, and occasionally one or two from respiratory collapse. Virtually all show extensive atherosclerosis ("hardening of the arteries") at autopsy. On the other hand, as Martin and many others have pointed out, there are many features seen in normal aging that are absent in HGPS. The metabolism of HG progerics, and in particular the function of the numerous proteins required to operate the body's various metabolic systems, seem quite normal for their true calendar age, and do not reflect the changes seen in the metabolism of the elderly. Their vision and hearing are excellent. Moreover, they experience none of the senile dementia common in older adults, and they have normal neurological function throughout life. Cancer, so common in the true elderly, is absent in HGPS.

Clearly there is something terribly wrong in these children. But what? What could possibly explain this bizarre and tragic compression of a human life into a handful of years? The marked uniformity of symptoms expressed in progerics suggests a common underlying disease mechanism. But what kind of a disease could account for what we see unfolding in these children? And what, if anything, can it tell us about the normal aging process?

One powerful piece of evidence that the aging process as manifested in these patients is connected to senescence as studied in other systems comes from analysis of their fibroblasts growing in vitro. In a study published in 1971, it was shown that skin-derived fibroblasts from HGPS children, when cultured in vitro, grew much more slowly than such fibroblasts taken from other children in the same family, and even more slowly than fibroblasts taken from their parents. In fact, doublings were scarcely detectable. Not only does the skin look old, its component cells behave as if they were old. By the criterion of replicative senescence, the HGPS children appeared to be even older than their parents.

By virtually any definition, HGPS is a disease, and it is a disease unlikely to be caused by external agents. By exclusion, we can confidently expect that it is ultimately explicable in terms of a genetic derangement, a mutation in one or more genes affecting one or more critical proteins. The question then becomes, how does this genetic defect arise? Is it a sporadic mutational event occurring in the lifetime of the afflicted individual, or is it inherited? Is it a dominant mutation, or is it recessive? Is it autosomal, or is it sex-linked? Questions like these are normally answered by following the disease in succeeding generations of families. Because there are so few HGPS individuals alive at any given time, and because they do not produce children who could inherit the disease, these questions are more difficult to resolve, but there are a number of things we can say about its genetic pattern. Since it affects both males and females equally, it is clearly autosomal and not sex-linked. Its extreme rarity could be consistent with a sporadic autosomal dominant mutation arising in a mature germ cell of one parent. This is rendered unlikely by the fact that there are several well-documented cases of more than one child in a single family with HGPS. We would then have to imagine that this rare mutation occurred spontaneously more than once in the parents of such families. From the limited information at hand, it seems most likely that HGPS represents an autosomal recessive genetic disease, in which both parents must be carriers of the defective gene. We do not yet know the identity of the gene (or genes) which, when mutated, can cause such a complex and devastating disease. But that a single genetic error can cause diseases of this type is suggested by another disorder on Martin's list: Werner's syndrome.

Werner's Syndrome

Werner's syndrome is named for Otto Werner, who first described this condition in his thesis for the M.D. degree in Germany in 1904, the same year that Gilford described his first patient. Like the Hutchinson-Gilford syndrome, this is clearly a progerial disorder, in which affected individuals experience some form of an accelerated aging process. It is nearly as rare; only about 200 cases have been described to date. But Werner's syndrome is without doubt distinct from HGPS. In his original report, Werner described four siblings with essentially identical symptoms: growth retardation, general atrophy of muscle and connective tissues, an aged appearance due to graying hair and wrinkled skin, and crippling joint deformities. But unlike HGPS, the onset of definitive symptoms in Werner's syndrome (WS) rarely begins before age twenty. Affected individuals seem perfectly normal as children, but they generally stop growing early in the adolescent years. Men are rarely more than five feet tall, with women several inches shorter. The average age of death in Werner's patients is forty-four years.

The accumulation of additional patients since Werner's time has allowed a clearer picture of the symptoms defining this disease. Hair graying and loss is one of the earlier symptoms, beginning, like growth retardation, during the adolescent years. It is usually not as complete as in HGPS. Secondary sexual hair develops reasonably normally in many cases, but may be lost as the syndrome progresses. During this period as well, patients start to display prematurely aged skin, although not as extensively as individuals with HGPS. The skin of the feet and hands is particularly affected, exhibiting the thin, dry, pigmented condition seen in HGPS, but also including the development of very thick calluses that sometimes ulcerate and even bleed. Facial skin also seems very old in appearance, due to loss of subcutaneous fat and nutritive cell layers. On the other hand skin in the trunk region is only minimally affected.

There is also a general wasting of muscle tissue in the extremities, accompanied by loss of bone mass, again with reasonable maintenance of both of these parameters in the trunk. The overall appearance is thus of small, old-looking limbs appended to a robust, young-looking trunk. The joints are often thickened and calcified, making movements difficult and painful. One of the most distinctive features of WS is the development of cataracts. Normally seen only in persons over fifty, cataracts develop in nearly all WS patients over thirty, setting in as early as ten years of age in a few individuals. The cataracts usually affect both eyes simultaneously. Other eye problems associated with old age are also common in these individuals.

As in HGPS, WS patients develop cardiovascular problems that are a common cause of death, although in those afflicted with WS there is a more generalized problem with occluded blood vessels that can lead to gangrene and limb amputation. This could be due to the fact that WS patients live longer. This longer survival may also account for other differences between Werner's and HGPS patients, such as the occurrence of maturity-onset (type II) diabetes and certain cancers in WS patients in the third and fourth decades of life; cancer is also a common cause of death in WS. Although somewhat sexually underdeveloped, individuals with this disease are in fact often fertile, and a number have reproduced. As with HGPS patients, fibroblasts taken from persons afflicted with WS show greatly reduced growth in vitro, comparable to fibroblasts taken from very old persons.

Studies with fibroblasts from WS patients have provided insight into the types of changes that occur in these cells as they age, and these changes appear to parallel those seen during normal aging. Fibroblasts (which are scattered throughout the entire body, especially in skin) are one of a number of cell types that produce a protein called collagen. Collagen is well known as the soft precursor substance of bones, laid down in embryos and newborns and later fortified by calcium into classical hard bone. But collagen plays a much wider role in the body, in the form of something called extracellular matrix, a semi-rigid, lattice-like structure to which cells adhere, and which gives tissues and organs their shape. Without collagen and extracellular matrix, the body would likely collapse down into a mass of tissue hanging from a skeletal frame. The collagen secreted by fibroblasts is used to make up this extracellular matrix. But fibroblasts are also capable of producing the enzyme collagenase, which degrades collagen. As fibroblasts senesce, either in vitro or in vivo, they switch from a collagen-producing to a collagenase-secreting (collagen-degrading) cell phenotype. Destruction of the extracellular matrix by fibroblasts could certainly cause many of the features associated with aging, such as wrinkled and sagging skin, and possibly some of the apparent wasting in muscle tissue.

A significant number of WS patients are born to consanguinous parents, particularly in Japan where first- and second-cousin marriages are more common than in the West; about three-quarters of all WS cases have been reported from Japan. The fact that WS occurs more frequently in consanguinous marriages, and affects offspring of both sexes, indicates that it is an autosomal recessive defect. About one in 5000 persons is estimated to carry the WS gene, leading to the appearance of WS in about one in 25 million births. Determining exactly *which* autosomal gene is defective in WS has been somewhat easier to approach than was the case for HGPS. Patients live longer, and occasionally even have offspring to whom the gene is passed. There is also a reasonable number of cases where more than one child is afflicted in the same family, which further supports the case for autosomal recessiveness and greatly helps in tracing the chromosomal location of genes.

A close study of the inheritance pattern of WS in Japan and in the United States traced the underlying gene to the short arm of chromosome 8. Using advanced techniques for gene mapping at the DNA level,* the chromosomal location of the WS gene was determined with sufficient accuracy to allow the very first isolation and sequencing of an apparent aging-associated gene, described in a joint Japanese-U.S. report published in April 1996. When the DNA sequence for the WS gene was converted into an amino-acid sequence and compared with other known sequences, the resulting 1,432-amino-acid protein looked very much like an enzyme called DNA helicase. This enzyme is so named because it plays a role in unwinding the two strands of DNA that form the DNA double helix (Fig. 5.2.) Once the gene was cloned, and the corresponding protein produced artificially, its identity as a DNA helicase was confirmed by direct testing for helicase activity. This is an exciting finding, because one of the major theories of aging

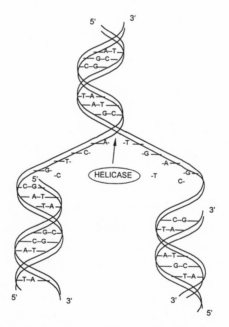

Figure 5.2. DNA unwinding under the influence of helicase during DNA replication.

---

*For a discussion of the methods used to map, isolate and clone human disease-associated genes, see William R. Clark, *The New Healers: The Promise and Problems of Molecular Medicine in the Twenty-First Century* (New York: Oxford University Press, 1997).

is that it results from the inability either to read, repair, or replicate DNA. While helicases themselves are not involved directly in any of these functions, they prepare the DNA for all three. And WS patients show extensive DNA abnormalities in their final decade of life.

But how could a defect in a single gene cause such a complex and specific set of symptoms, many of which mimic closely some of the phenotypes of aging, such as replicative senescence of fibroblasts in vitro? This is the question now occupying the new breed of doctors and scientists who look at human health at the level of molecular genetics. The answer may lie in a fact about genes discussed in the last chapter. The majority of our genes—the so-called housekeeping genes—are expressed in every cell in the body. A mutation in a single housekeeping gene, which may play basically the same role in cells throughout the body, may have a sharply different impact in different tissues, depending largely on the special-function genes and gene products with which it interacts in those cells and tissues. DNA helicases could certainly be considered housekeeping genes. A mutation in the ability to unwind DNA may play out differently in different cells and tissues. But before we try to refine this answer in greater detail, let us look at yet another aging syndrome in which a quite similar type of gene may very well be involved.

Cockayne Syndrome

Another rare type of progeria, first detected in a brother-sister pair, was described in England by E. A. Cockayne in 1936. He did not classify these cases as progerias at first; the title of both his initial paper and a follow-up report was "Dwarfism with Retinal Atrophy and Deafness." Over the decade following his second report, other cases were identified with the same symptoms, and a closer following of affected individuals showed that they, too, were experiencing at least some facets of an accelerated aging process. Cockayne syndrome (CS) soon took its place along with HGPS and WS as one of the principal progerias. The dwarfism, deafness, and blindness noted by Cockayne are still hallmarks of this condition. The children seem perfectly normal during the first year or two of life. Growth retardation and slowness to speak and comprehend normal language become of increasing concern in the third year, although some cases are not fully recognized until the fifth or sixth year. Both males and females are very small in stature, rarely reaching more than four feet in height. There are some of the same skin and muscle tissue atrophy problems seen in HGPS and WS, the same difficulties with occluded joints, and the same progressive thinning of the bones. Sexual development is also retarded. As in HGPS, afflicted individuals rarely live beyond their early twenties. However, CS patients do not show many of the features of the other two progerias, and have several quite distinctive features of their own (Table 5.2). For example, there is no noticeable atherosclerosis, and no cardiovascular disease in CS patients; on the other hand, there is progressive degeneration of central nervous system tissues, which may be related to the loss of sight and hearing functions. CS patients die of neurological degeneration rather than heart failure. Of great interest to gerontologists, many of the changes seen in the brain at autopsy closely parallel those seen in normal humans beyond the seventh decade or so of life. Whether or not CS patients undergo true senile dementia or not is unclear; they are often quite retarded in mental development because of blindness and loss of hearing, which makes assessment of mental function difficult.

One of the most characteristic features of Cockayne syndrome is an unusual sensitivity of the skin to ultraviolet light. This symptom, missing in the other progerias we have discussed, is also one of the hallmarks of the normal aging process in humans, and is thought to be related to a progressive loss of the ability to repair light-induced damage to DNA. There is some evidence that a helicase defect may be involved in CS as well. Since only cells at the very surface of the body are exposed to ultraviolet light, this obviously is not a cause of aging in tissues other than skin. However, the inability to repair DNA generally may reflect a deeper problem that could have major implications for senescence. We now know that cells constantly monitor their DNA for irregularities, and have several mechanisms for restoring any changes that might creep into inherited DNA sequences throughout the life of the organism. "Normal" mutational events—those that do not alter the basic chemical nature of the DNA itself, and which might give rise to useful new forms of genes—are not corrected by these repair mechanisms. However, mutations such as those caused by radiation, certain mutagenic chemicals, or even some of the highly oxidative molecules that are by-products of normal cellular metabolism can

Table 5.2. *A Comparison of normal aging and accelerated aging in various progerias*

Feature	Normal Aging	Hutchinson–Gilford progeria	Werner syndrome	Cockayne syndrome
Hair loss	Sixth decade	First year	Second decade	Some body hair loss
Skin changes	Global; fourth decade	Global; first year	Extremities only; second decade	Moderate
Atherosclerosis	Fourth decade	First decade	Second decade	Absent
Cataracts	Sixth decade	Absent	Third decade	Absent
Sexual development	Second decade	Absent; no reproduction	Moderate; second decade; reproduction possible	Slight; no reproduction
Maturity-onset (type II) diabetes	Fifth decade	Absent	Fourth decade	Absent
Senile dementia	Eighth decade	Absent	Mild or absent	Second decade (some aspects)
Cancer	Common after fifth decade	Absent	Common after third decade	Absent
U.V. sensitivity	Sixth decade	Absent	Absent	Common from birth

cause distortions in the structure of the DNA itself, and are readily detected and corrected by excising the distorted region and filling it in with unaltered building blocks.

Defects in the ability to repair DNA damage are known to be the cause of yet another genetic disease called xeroderma pigmentosum (XP). Persons afflicted with XP do not normally experience problems with accelerated aging, but like WS patients they are extremely sensitive to ultraviolet light. It turns out that mutations in any one of about seven different genes—all presumably involved in DNA repair—can cause XP. One of these genes was recently shown to encode a helicase-like molecule. Whether it is the same as the helicase molecule in WS is unclear at present, but it is interesting that this is the one XP gene that, when mutant, causes CS-like symptoms. And yet another genetic disorder with ultraviolet light sensitivity and some features of a progeria—Bloom syndrome—was shown in mid-1996 to be caused by a faulty helicase-like gene. We will explore the possible involvement of defective DNA repair mechanisms in senescence and cancer in more detail in later chapters.

The progerias in themselves have by no means solved the riddle of aging and senescence. Some have argued that they do not reflect the true aging process at all. In none of them do we see all of the phenotypes of human aging, and in some a particular phenotype may differ slightly from "normal" aging. We even see some changes that are not thought to be part of the aging process at all. But so-called normal aging is itself highly variable; what we define as the norm is itself only an average of all the individual phenotypes we have seen. The aging events taking place in each of the progerias may well represent only a restricted portion of a given "normal" aging process. The diseases discussed here are all single-gene defects; no one ever claimed that aging is caused by a single gene, so it is not surprising that these segmental progerias do not display the full range of aging defects. Nevertheless, they reveal several important things that we should bear in mind as we proceed through the following chapters.

First, we see in the progerias that variations in a single gene can have far-reaching effects in terms of the phenotypes of aging. This would not be predicted by theories of senescence that postulate the random accumulation over evolutionary time of senescence-related genes in different species. Proponents of these theories would expect large numbers of different aging genes, each affecting a different tissue in a different way. Thus mutations in no single one of these genes would be expected to have more than a local effect, causing accelerated aging in a restricted number of cells or tissues. Perhaps that may account for some of the resistance to accepting the progerias as reflective of the true aging process. Looking at the progerias, however, it is not at all difficult to imagine that a relatively small number of genes, probably housekeeping genes, could account for most if not all of the aging phenotypes.

The progerias also make it clear that the aging process per se in humans is not rigidly time-dependent. Changes that would normally take sixty or seventy years to manifest in the normal aging process—hearts or kidneys wearing out, skin becoming thin and discolored—are brought to completion in a decade or so in HGPS. These hearts did not cave in from a lifetime of physical exertion; the skin did not age from years of exposure to the sun. These changes are thus unlikely to be caused directly by a "wearing- out" process per se. In terms of a three-gene scenario for senescence, what we could be seeing in the progerias is either a defect in senescence repressor genes or a malfunction in senescence regulator genes. Defective senescence repressor genes might result in gene products unable to prevent or repair damage caused by senescence effector genes, allowing senescent damage to accumulate at an accelerated rate. Defects in senescence regulator genes might result in an earlier than normal turn-off of senescence repressor genes, allowing senescence to begin ahead of schedule.

As far as we know, all of the progerias are caused by a defect—a harmful allelic variation—in a single gene. Each of these allelic variants is able to induce a broad range of the symptoms associated with normal aging phenotype. We must remember that these may not be the variants associated with the normal aging process. But what the progerias suggest is that the genes that these alleles represent are excellent candidates for genes involved in a fundamental way in the aging process. Increasingly, these appear to be genes involved in causing damage to DNA or in repairing that damage.

Aging is almost certainly, as George Martin guessed twenty years ago, a multigenic process. As we will see in coming chapters, a number of "normal" genes have already been proposed as candidates that contribute to aging late in life. It is sometimes assumed that the total number of these "gerontogenes" must be quite large, based on the complexity of the aging phenotype and on the many genes already under investigation. On the other hand, the incredible spectrum of aging-like phenotypic changes wrought in the single-gene progerias suggests that the actual number of such genes may not have to be terribly large.

6

Cycling to Senescence

Few discoveries have rocked the generally staid world of gerontology research quite like the pronouncement of Leonard Hayflick and Paul Moorehead in their 1961 paper, "The Serial Cultivation of Human Diploid Cell Strains." It had been dogma for nearly fifty years that cells removed from the body would grow virtually forever in vitro. This directed the attention of everyone interested in aging away from the cell itself and toward factors within the body that caused otherwise immortal cells to age and die. But Hayflick and Moorehead showed otherwise. And they provided convincing evidence that the aging of cells in vitro—replicative senescence, as it came to be called—was a reasonably good reflection of cellular aging in vivo.

With the verification of their finding by others (which took a few years, given the entrenched belief in the inherent immortality of isolated cells), the cell became a primary focus of aging researchers everywhere. But the initial rush of enthusiasm was soon tempered by some serious questions. What is the relation of replicative senescence in vitro to aging of the organism? Could the phenomenon of replicative senescence be an ultimate cause of aging, or is it simply a reflection of some broader underlying process controlling cellular senescence generally? This latter question was prompted by the fact that a very large proportion of the body's cells divide very little, and in some cases not at all, during the lifetime of an adult organism.

Nevertheless, a great deal of excitement was generated by the clear demonstration that, like their primitive eukaryotic ancestors from whom they are separated by billions of years of evolution, mammalian cells grown in vitro undergo progressive changes in size and shape, accompanied by a gradual slowing and then cessation of cell division. Moreover, mammalian cells in culture also pass through a series of internal biochemical changes that mimic rather closely changes seen in mammalian cells aging in vivo. The total number of in vitro cell divisions—the replicative lifespan—is genetically fixed for each species, and, intriguingly, the replicative lifespan characteristic of a particular species correlates with its maximum potential lifespan; cells from species with longer maximum lifespans undergo a greater number of total cell divisions in vitro, starting with cells taken from the embryo. Moreover, as individuals proceed through their lifespan, the number of divisions their cells are capable of in vitro decreases; cells taken from very old individuals (and, in the case of humans, younger individuals with a premature aging syndrome) divide only a few times in vitro before entering a senescent state.

A great deal has been made of the variability of these numbers within and between species. They are admittedly not very precise, partly because the number of times any cell will divide in vitro is easily perturbed by slight changes in growth conditions. Different labs will thus come up with different values. But all investigators have found that if the completion of a eukaryotic cell division program is interrupted, either naturally by cyst formation or artificially by freezing the cells, the program will resume pretty much where it left off once the cells are returned to a fully active metabolic state. It seems that even human cells, at least those that actively divide during their lifetime, appear to have retained the primitive eukaryotic characteristic of determining lifespan in terms of an approximate total number of cell divisions, rather than by absolute calendar reckoning.

But how do cells know when the clock has run out, when they have completed their "Hayflick limit"? How do cells count? The key to understanding how cells could "know" how many cell divisions they have undergone, and how cells could switch from active division to a state of senescence, lies in an understanding of something called the eukaryotic cell cycle. The cell cycle is the complete sequence of events that leads to mitosis, in which a single parental cell gives rise to two daughter cells, normally identical in every way to the parent. During the cell cycle, the DNA must be faithfully replicated, and then the cell must physically divide in two, apportioning the existing cell organelles along with the DNA into the new daughter cells. The daughters then must replenish their stock of organelles and other cellular constituents before they are ready to begin another round of cell replication.

All of this happens in a series of closely regulated molecular events that collectively constitute the cell cycle (Fig. 6.1). It is among these molecular events that we must look for clues to cellular time keeping and for the basis of replicative senescence. The cells that make up multicellular organisms like ourselves do not divide spontaneously or capriciously; they divide only in response to signals coming to them from the outside (extracellular) environment. A cell that has not recently been dividing will be in what is called the G_0 (resting) stage of the cycle. When an appropriate signal to divide (a growth signal) is

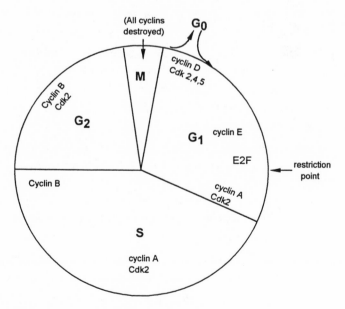

Figure 6.1. The mammalian cell cycle.

received at the cell surface, the cell passes from G_0 to the G_1 (growth 1) stage, and then on into the S (synthesis) stage, where it begins to synthesize DNA. To facilitate this process of DNA replication, each of the chromosomes housing the DNA loosens up and the double-stranded DNA molecule, under guidance from a DNA helicase, unwinds into single strands. When the process of DNA replication is complete, the cell passes into G_2, where it now has double the normal amount of DNA. Cells usually pass rather quickly through G_2 to reach M, the mitotic phase of the cell cycle, where the physical process of cell division and apportioning of cell contents takes place. When mitosis is completed, if the extracellular growth signal that caused the G_0 cells to enter G_1 in the first place is still present, the cells will proceed from M directly into G_1 and another round of cell division. If this signal is lacking, the cells will return to G_0. In either case, the cells will have returned to a normal diploid amount of DNA.

Much of the information we have about how cells are guided through a complete cell cycle has been obtained by studying developmental events in frog eggs and analyzing cell division in yeast cells. Yeast cells in particular have a number of advantages for such studies: They have a very rapid cell cycle time (90 minutes, versus about 20 hours for most mammalian cells), and we know a great deal about the genes in yeast and what they do. Of course frog eggs and yeast cells are very different from human cells, and we might wonder what we could learn from studying them that would help us understand ourselves. But as it turns out, the process of cell division is very strongly conserved in evolution, and in fact nearly everything we have learned about the cell cycle in these two systems has proved to be almost directly applicable to the replication of human cells.

Let's begin our journey through the cycle G_0. Cells in G_0 have left the cell cycle after their previous mitosis, and are not dividing; they will do so only when they receive growth signals from outside the cell telling them to reenter active cell division. Animal cells respond to a wide range of physical and chemical signals produced in their environment. They can be directed to divide (or to stop dividing) by direct physical contact with surrounding cells, through membrane-membrane interactions. More commonly, such signals are received in the form of free-floating chemical messages—growth signals—that arrive through the bloodstream. These messages come from other cells, including those in the brain or in various hormone-producing tissues and organs. These small molecular messengers, which are often (but not always) proteins, bind to specific receptors on the surface of the targeted cell.

When a growth factor arrives at a cell surface and binds to its specific receptor, the receptor transmits a signal through the membrane to intracellular "second messengers." A string of these messengers passes the signal along until it finally reaches the nucleus and its ultimate target, the DNA. Most growth signals result in the "switching on" of new genes in the DNA that will carry out the functions called forth by the growth signal, including synthesis of the DNA itself. These new genes are first transcribed into messenger RNA, which leaves the nucleus and proceeds to the cellular machinery specialized in making proteins. There, the messages are translated into the protein encoded in the transcribed gene. Once a growth signal has been received and the cell has been brought into G_1, it begins its journey through the rest of the cell cycle. Continuous interaction of the growth factor with the surface receptor is necessary throughout about the first 80 percent or so of G_1; however, once the cell has reached the so-called restriction point in G_1, the cell will proceed through the rest of the cell cycle in the absence of external growth factor.

The cell is guided through G_1 and subsequent cell-cycle phases by several distinct types of proteins. One set of molecules, the cyclins and the cyclin-dependent kinases (Cdks), are synthesized very early in G_1 in response to the incoming growth signal. A cyclin protein combines with a Cdk protein to form a dimeric molecule; at different stages of the cell cycle, as we shall see, different cyclins interact with different Cdks to create unique, stage-specific protein complexes. The function of these different complexes is to activate the cellular machinery necessary to complete a particular stage of the cell cycle. In some cases, this may involve interaction of the dimer with yet other proteins, present in the cell but held in an inactive state, so that they can perform their own stage-specific functions, such as DNA replication in S phase, or any of the various steps in mitosis such as pulling the replicated chromosomes apart or actually dividing the cell in two. In other cases, the cyclin-Cdk dimers interact with DNA and participate in the induction of new, stage-specific genes and proteins needed to carry out stage-specific functions. A second set of molecules, referred to collectively as E2F, plays a very important role later in G_1. E2F interacts directly with the DNA to help transcribe genes whose products will be necessary for the G_1 to S transition. The successful activation of E2F marks the restriction point, where the cell becomes independent of continued external growth signal stimulation for proceeding through the rest of the cell cycle.

None of these proteins are present in cells resting in the G_0 state. All are formed only after the cell receives an appropriate growth signal. Cyclin D is formed very quickly as the cell enters G_1, and interacts with Cdk molecules 2, 4, and 5—also formed very shortly after receipt of a proliferation signal—to move the cell forward to the point where it is ready to begin the all-important step of DNA synthesis. At that point (referred to as the "G_1/S interface"), the level of cyclin E has built up in the cell to a level where it begins to compete for the Cdk2 molecules. The new cyclin E-Cdk2 complexes push the cell across the G_1/S interface and into the true S phase.

Soon the level of cyclin A starts to build up in the cell, and this cyclin begins competing for the scarce Cdk2 molecules; the resulting cyclin A-Cdk2 complexes activate the cellular proteins actually involved in DNA synthesis. There is good evidence that cyclin A-Cdk2 may be part of a group of proteins that unwinds the DNA helices to prepare them for copying. This association of cyclins with a helicase activity may have important implications for senescence, as we shall see later. Once DNA synthesis is complete, and the cells are poised at the S/G_2 interface, cyclin B, which had been synthesized during the S and G_2 phases, starts to interact with the Cdk2 molecules and activates the machinery necessary to carry out mitosis. During mitosis, any remaining cell-cycling proteins are destroyed. As the cell leaves mitosis, if the growth signal is still present outside the cell, it will enter directly into G_1 and continue on through another cycle. If no signal is present, the cell will move into G_0 and cease cycling, because the cyclins and Cdk molecules needed to push the cell through G_1 are not there.

Regulation of the Cell Cycle

The cell cycle just described is subject to a number of controls to ensure that cellular proliferation occurs in response to proper external growth signals, and *only* in response to these signals. When cells enter into unstimulated or unscheduled proliferation, the result, in the absence of appropriate controls, may well be the development of cancer (see Chapter 7). Controls are also necessary to ensure that each stage is completed before entry into the following stage. For example, if a cell rushed into mitosis before synthesis of the DNA and reassembly of chromosomes was complete, the daughter cells would inherit garbled genetic information and would almost certainly be unable to function. A close study of the "checkpoints" located at strategic places in the cell cycle, where the cycle can be brought to an instant halt if all is not well, has provided important insights into cellular senescence, which is characterized by an inability of cells to divide.

Some of the checkpoints present in the normal cell cycle are shown in Figure 6.2. One of the most important checkpoints occurs in G_1, where the DNA that is about to be replicated in the S phase is examined for damage. The type of DNA damage that is of most concern at this stage is that caused either by radiation (presumably cosmic radiation would be the normal biological threat) or by chemicals, either environmental chemicals that manage to get inside the cell or chemical breakdown products arising from normal cellular metabolism. Particularly for cells that may have spent a long time in G_0 since the last cell division, there may be substantial cumulative damage of this type; damaged DNA could well contain mutated genes, and thus pose a serious threat to the organism.

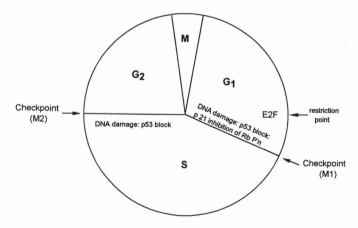

Figure 6.2. Checkpoints in the cell cycle.

Damage of this type is detected by one of the most important molecules in the cell cycle, called p53. (The p stands for "protein; 53 indicates that its size in atomic units is 53,000.) We do not know exactly how p53 recognizes damaged DNA, but we do know that when damage is detected, p53 brings the cell cycle to a screeching halt by inducing the synthesis of other molecules that inhibit the cyclin-Cdk complexes guiding the cell through G_1 into S. If the damage is particularly severe, and beyond repair, p53 may also instruct the cell to enter apoptosis—to start down the path to cellular suicide. Cells have a variety of DNA repair mechanisms; if the damage can be repaired, the p53-induced block is lifted, and if the cell has not reached a point of no return in the apoptotic pathway, it may be allowed to proceed on through the cycle. We will examine these processes in more detail in a moment, for they are also likely related to senescence.

There is a second checkpoint for DNA damage at the end of the S phase. Here, the DNA is examined for breaks in the DNA chains that might have occurred during DNA replication. Broken DNA would not segregate properly into daughter cells during mitosis, and thus if broken DNA is detected (probably by p53), the cells are arrested in G_2 until the breaks can be repaired. In a separate checkpoint toward the end of the S phase the DNA is examined to ensure that it has actually been replicated in its entirety; the cell cannot proceed into G_2 with unreplicated DNA present. At the very least one of the daughter cells would get shortchanged in terms of DNA received, and would be unable to survive. Exactly how this checkpoint operates is not understood at present. There are also safeguards to ensure that all of the DNA has been replicated only once during S phase. And finally, cells that have successfully exited from S phase cannot reenter S unless they have been through mitosis. The cyclin B present during G_2, which is normally lost in M, would prevent the cells from reentering S. All of these controls act to ensure that all of the DNA is replicated once, and only once, in each cell cycle. Cells are also able to detect whether the machinery for mitosis itself has been damaged.

What does "checkpoint" mean in molecular terms? How is progress through the cell cycle halted if all is not well? For most of the regulatory points discussed so far, the cell cycle appears to be disrupted by the production of proteins that bind to cyclin-Cdk complexes and inactivate them. For example, when p53 detects damaged DNA in G_1,

S, or G_2, it induces the formation of a special protein called p21, which binds to cyclin-Cdk dimers and blocks them from mediating their stage-specific functions. In particular, p21 prevents cyclin D-Cdk and cyclin E-Cdk from moving cells out of G_1 and into S. Human fibroblasts in which p21 has been damaged are unable to enter senescence on cue. Importantly, p21 does not block *all* DNA synthesis; damaged DNA can still be repaired in the presence of p21, and this repair often requires synthesis of short stretches of DNA. p21 has no effect on this "repair synthesis" of DNA; in fact, there is good evidence that repair synthesis is actively promoted by p21.

One of the more interesting and important negative regulators of the cell cycle is the retinoblastoma protein (Rb), originally discovered as a protein missing or mutated in the childhood cancer of that name. Rb was subsequently found to be missing or altered in a number of other cancers as well; we will discuss the role of Rb and similar molecules (including p53) in cancer generally in Chapter 7. In the normal cell cycle, Rb is present in the cell in an active form in the early G_1 phase, just up to the restriction point, at which time it is suddenly rendered inactive. When it is active, Rb binds tightly to the E2F family of molecules involved in transcriptional events in late G_1, preventing them from initiating transcription of genes needed for progress of the cell into S phase (Fig. 6.3). As cells approach the restriction point in G_1, cyclin D and E complexes formed with Cdk proteins 4 and 6 inactivate Rb, causing it to release its hold on E2F. The proteins necessary for S phase are now made by the cell, and further progress through the cycle becomes independent of external growth factors. Rb remains inactive throughout the rest of the cell cycle.

The Cell Cycle and Replicative Senescence

When cells age in vitro and eventually stop dividing, they arrest in G_1—not, as might be expected for permanently nondividing cells, in G_0. But unlike other cells in G_0 or G_1, senescent cells do not respond to normal growth signals by continuing on into S phase. The cells do not lose the ability to respond to all incoming signals; they selectively lose sensitivity to growth signals. One possibility for the failure to respond to growth signals could be that the machinery necessary to do so is not in place or has worn out and is no longer func-

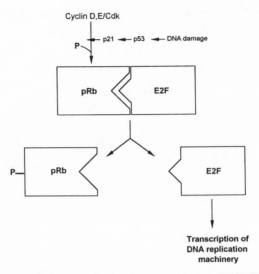

Figure 6.3. The interaction of the retinoblastoma protein with E2F. During early G₁, the E2F complex is bound up with the pRb protein and cannot initiate DNA synthesis (S phase). Normally, toward the end of G₁, the cyclin D,E/Cdk complex adds a P (phosphate group) to pRb, causing it to release E2F. However, in the presence of DNA damage, p53 and p21 are induced, blocking the phosphorylation step and hence preventing the cell from entering into S phase.

tional. But there is experimental evidence indicating that this explanation is unlikely. The receptors for the growth factors are still detectable on the cell surface, and the machinery necessary to process the signal inside the cell is intact.

An important clue to the nature of the defect in these cells comes from cell fusion experiments. It is possible to induce two individual cells to fuse into one; the resulting hybrid cell (called a heterokaryon) has two nuclei and two complete sets of all cellular components. When senescent cells are fused together with younger, actively dividing cells so that their internal contents can mix freely, the heterokaryon will have an ample supply of organelles and chemical components necessary for cell division from the younger cell partner, yet the heterokaryon remains senescent. As may be remembered from Chapter 2, the same thing happens when senescent and young yeast cells are fused together; senescence is a dominant trait. The simplest explanation of these results, in both yeast and humans, is that the senescent cell is senescent because it contains a soluble, diffusible, replication-inhibiting molecule inside the cell; when an older and younger cell are fused, the factor present in the older cell also represses any capacity for cell division the younger cell may have brought into the heterokaryon.

Several laboratories began a search for soluble factors present in senescent cells that could explain their failure to enter into S phase. One of the earliest findings was that the Rb protein in senescent cells remains present in the fully activated form. As just discussed, Rb is normally inactivated late in G_1, just at the restriction point, so that E2F can be released and participate in transcription of new gene products required for entry into S phase. The presence of active Rb protein, physically bound to E2F, could certainly explain the failure of senescent cells to progress into S phase, but seemed incompatible with the cell fusion experiments done earlier. Why wouldn't the younger cell fusion partner be able to inactivate the senescent cell partner's Rb proteins?

The answer became apparent upon backtracking further into G_1. As we have seen, Rb is ordinarily inactivated by cyclin-Cdk complexes (Fig. 6.3). But cyclin-Cdk complexes themselves can be inactivated by p21. And indeed, careful analysis of senescent human fibroblasts also showed a very high level of p21. The presence of this potent inhibitory molecule in senescent cells helped make sense of the cell fusion experiments and explained why senescence is a dominant trait. p21 molecules (and related inhibitory proteins called p16 and p24) contributed by the senescent fusion partner would exert a dominant inhibitory effect on the cyclin-Cdk complexes of *both* fusion partners, thus neutralizing the ability of these complexes to inactivate Rb, which would continue to exert its suppressive effect on E2F.

The key role played by p21 in this process supplies an important clue to the nature of the underlying force driving replicative senescence. p21, remember, is induced by p53, and as far as we know the only thing that p53 responds to is damaged DNA. That suggests that damaged DNA is a major cause of replicative senescence. p53 can shunt a cell into a senescent state at any time, should it encounter damaged DNA. But the data all point to an accumulation, over the normal replicative lifetime of dividing cells, of DNA damage that eventually pushes the cell into senescence. We will examine in just a moment exactly what the sources of this damaged DNA may be.

The foregoing model suggests ways in which it should be possible to bypass replicative senescence in vitro. The critical block at G_1/S is caused by a failure of Rb to release E2F. If the Rb-E2F complex could be dissociated by artificial means, then the senescent cells should be able to proceed into S phase in response to appropriate growth signals. This has actually been achieved in mouse and rat fibroblasts using a virus called simian virus 40 (SV40). If mouse fibroblasts are infected with SV40 prior to completion of their replicative limit, the cells will continue to divide well beyond their normal limit. An analysis of this effect showed that SV40 encodes a protein called T antigen that can disrupt the interaction of Rb and E2F. In cells in which cyclin-Cdk complexes are inhibited by p21 and related molecules, simply the introduction of the T antigen gene, by itself, is sufficient to relieve the G_1/S block imposed by Rb—the rest of the virus is unnecessary. In this form of individual cell "gene therapy," the gene is taken up by the cell and transcribed and translated as if it were part of the cell's own genome. The resulting T antigen protein then binds to Rb, forcing it to release E2F. T antigen also binds to p53, thus decreasing the concentration of p21 in the cell.

Other viruses were shown to do the same thing—adenovirus, for example, uses proteins called E1A and E1B to bypass normal blocks to cell division; the human papilloma virus that causes warts uses proteins called E6 and E7. The ability of viruses to do this is simply part of a larger strategy that viruses employ for their own purposes. In bypassing the normal controls on cellular proliferation, viruses essentially create an immortal host for themselves, where they can reproduce their own kind without worrying about the cell becoming uncooperatively senescent. Simply bypassing the G_1/S block is probably not sufficient for achieving true immortality, however. Most virally infected cells that pass through the G_1/S barrier (sometimes called the "M1," or "mortality 1," barrier) apparently get trapped, particularly in human cells, at a second barrier (M2) further on in the cell cycle. This second barrier puts the potentially immortal cells in a state of crisis; only a few cells emerge from M2, but those that do are truly immortal and capable of indefinite cell division.

Interestingly, studies with SV40 suggest that cells transformed by a virus or a particular viral gene do not lose track of time on the cell cycle clock. If the T antigen gene is turned off in mouse cells before the infected cell has reached its limiting number of cell divisions, the cells will proceed to the limiting number and then enter senescence, right on schedule. If left in place, the T antigen can carry the cell beyond its natural number of cell divisions, but in that case the moment the T antigen gene is turned off the cell will immediately enter a senescent state.

Another verification of the proposed model comes from experiments in which a gene encoding E2F itself was introduced into mouse cells in a senescence-like state called quiescence. The introduced gene was able to direct the production of an amount of E2F in excess of the active Rb molecules present; the excess E2F allowed the cells to proceed through into S phase. (This provides, incidentally, an elegant proof that the replicative machinery in a senescent cell is still functionally intact.) The molecular elements of replicative senescence are thus seen to be nothing more than a special application of the checkpoint mechanisms already in place to prevent unscheduled cell division, for example, cancer.

In humans, these same mechanisms participate in effecting cellular senescence, but there may be additional mechanisms as well. Human fibroblasts are notoriously difficult to immortalize in vitro with viruses. SV40 infection will often extend the replicative lifespan for ten or twenty doublings, but then the cells usually become senescent; they appear to make it through M1, but cannot get past M2. Moreover, infection of even mouse fibroblasts with SV40 or the gene for T antigen, once they are fully senescent, can help them get into S phase, but they never make it through to mitosis. Something apparently happens to cells once they settle into the senescent state that makes it difficult to draw them back out into cell division; it is as if they underwent some final step in differentiation, making a subsequent switch to any other state impossible. In human cells there is good reason to believe there may be additional barriers to unwanted cell divisions in later parts of the cell cycle such as G_2/M, as well as at the G_1/S interface.

How Do Cells Keep Time?

Replicative senescence in vitro offers one of the clearest looks yet available at the molecular mechanisms underlying at least one type of cellular senescence. Yet the picture remains incomplete. One point that is not entirely clear concerns the nature of the internal clock that tells dividing cells when they have reached their replicative limit. How do cells count cell cycles, and know when they are approaching their limiting number of cell divisions in vitro, maintaining this ability even in the presence of an overriding proliferation-inducing virus? One reasonable guess is that a portion of the inhibitory molecules that form the checkpoint apparatus are carried forward after each round of cell division, gradually accumulating until they reach a level that simply blocks cell division without any particular alarm being raised in the cell. All of the inhibitory events discussed thus far can be traced back to p21, which may accumulate as the cell cycles progress.

In early rounds of cell division, we imagine that such inhibitory molecules would reach these levels only if "super-induced" by some sort of accident—damage to the DNA, for example, or incorrect or incomplete DNA synthesis. The cyclins and Cdk molecules that drive the cell cycle are destroyed after each cycle, during mitosis. Inhibitory molecules like p21 are not destroyed, as far as we know, although they would be partitioned into the two daughter cells at the end of each cycle, cutting their effective concentration in half. Nevertheless, if a reasonably full complement of inhibitors is synthesized with each cell cycle, they might well continue to increase over time, and at some point a cell will be unable to respond to normal growth signals by dividing because the cyclins and Cdks that are induced by growth signals will simply be overwhelmed by preexisting inhibitors. Infection with a virus like SV40 or adenovirus could overcome these increased levels for a time, but even then at some point the increased levels of internal inhibitors may overwhelm viral proteins. And of course p21, as we have said, is ultimately controlled by p53, so it is possible that what happens with succeeding cycles is a gradual increase in p21 accumulation through increased p53 activity, rather than a decrease in p21 destruction. Intriguingly, p53 is also expressed at high levels in senescent human fibroblasts.

But does the accumulation of these molecules just happen stochastically throughout the life of the cell, or could it be driven and controlled by specific intracellular events? The major role of p53 and p21 seems to be in detecting and controlling DNA damage. Is there some systematic, cycle-dependent event happening inside cells that results in cumulative DNA damage? Recent research into this question has uncovered what is perhaps the best candidate yet for the internal clock that tells cells when they have reached their replicative limit: telomeres.

When single-cell life forms made the transition from prokaryotes to eukaryotes several billion years ago, a number of important changes occurred in the way cells manage their DNA. First, they put DNA inside a nucleus, where its environment could be controlled more precisely. Proteins and other chemicals needed to read and repair DNA could now be concentrated around the DNA itself, rather than being spread throughout the entire cell. A second important change that occurred was an increase in the total amount of DNA per cell. Eukaryotes are much more complex than prokaryotes, and require many more kinds of genes to operate the cell. Thus, whereas prokaryotes had only a single chromosome, eukaryotes began dividing their DNA into multiple chromosomes; humans, for example, have 23 different kinds of chromosomes. Moreover, eukaryotes became diploid, keeping two copies of every chromosome instead of one. One major advantage of diploidy is that every gene is present in two copies; if one copy is damaged or mutated and unable to function, the other copy can carry the cell along. Humans thus have 46 chromosomes, or 23 pairs.

Another change that occurred in the way DNA was kept in cells involved its linearization. Prokaryotes all keep their single chromosome in closed circular form; eukaryotes introduced a single double-strand cut in the circle to make their chromosomes linear. But this created a problem. The open ends of chromosomes are rather sticky; multiple linear chromosomes in a cell could clump together in a variety of bizarre ways that would greatly interfere with their ability to function, and that would make them almost impossible to replicate during the cell cycle. The tendency of randomly broken chromosome ends to adhere to other chromosomes is a common cause of cancer, as we shall see. Eukaryotes solved this problem (presumably, simultaneously with chromosomal linearization) by developing structures to "cap" each end of the open chromosome (Fig. 6.4). These are the structures called telomeres. Telomeres consist of short motifs of DNA repeated over and over at the tips of each chromosome. The human motif is TTAGGG, repeated 1500 to 2000 times. The telomeric caps also protect the open ends of chromosomes from digestion by enzymes. At some point, eukaryotes also began using telomeres to anchor the chromosomes to the nuclear membrane, which seems to be important for efficient chromosomal functioning.

Because of the way that DNA is replicated during each S phase, the

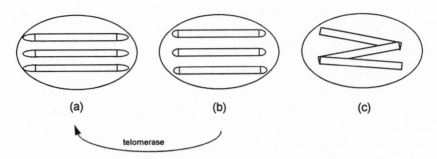

Figure 6.4. Telomere loss (*A, B*), if not restored by telomerase, can lead to chromosomal clumping (*C*).

terminal motif units defining each telomere are not copied during each round of cell division. In fact, a number of motif units are lost from the end of each chromosome after each round of DNA replication. In many single-cell eukaryotes that divide extensively as a normal part of their life cycle, there is a special enzyme called telomerase that can restore the telomeric ends to chromosomes. Telomerase is also detectable in multicellular eukaryotes, but only in the ovaries and testes (although not in mature sperm and ova) and in cells of the early, rapidly dividing embryo. It is also present in cells of the body that must continue to divide throughout most of the life cycle: hair follicle cells, certain gut cells, and white blood cells, for example. However, this enzyme is either absent or found at extremely low levels in most adult somatic cells of higher eukaryotes under normal conditions. It has thus been proposed that telomeres could be an important part of an internal clock mechanism, at least for dividing cells.

With each round of cell division, more and more of the protective telomeric cap would be lost from each chromosome, until at some point chromosomes would perhaps detach from the nuclear membrane or even begin to clump together. Detachment of the chromosomes would make it very difficult to "read" them for purposes of converting genes into proteins. More important, exposed regions of DNA within these detached chromosomes could be interpreted as damaged DNA. Certainly if the chromosomes clump together, duplicating them properly during the cell cycle would be virtually impossible. Finally, damaged DNA exposed either in incompleted teleomeric tips or as a result of induced chromosomal abnormalities could activate the p53-p21 damage control system and bring the cell cycle to a halt. So telomere shortening is a very attractive possibility for explaining replicative senescence.

Telomeres can indeed be observed to shorten throughout the life-span of cultured human fibroblasts, and in the cells of humans as they age in vivo. The average telomere length of fibroblasts at the time they are placed into culture in vitro is in fact a better predictor of how many doublings they will undergo than is the age of the fibroblast donor. Telomeres are significantly shorter in HGPS and WS patients than in age-matched controls. And chromosomal clumping has actually been observed in very old human cells in vivo and in human fibroblasts as they approach senescence in vitro. Like the rest of the DNA in the nucleus, telomeres are susceptible to damage, and the ability to repair this damage has been shown to decline with age. The accumulation of telomere damage, along with a cycle-dependent shortening, could at some point very well induce the type of DNA abnormalities detected by p53. It has also been proposed that reinduction of telomerase activity may be one critical barrier (M2 or beyond) to the complete transformation of somatic cells by viruses; fully immortalized cells have the longer telomeres characteristic of germ cells or embryonic cells, suggesting telomerase activity has been restored.

The possibility that telomeres are the internal clock that counts cell divisions is an extremely intriguing one. It is consistent with everything we understand about how the cell cycle is regulated, and in particular how it is brought to a halt. However, until very recently there was considerable doubt about whether telomere shortening is a primary cause of replicative senescence, a result of replicative senescence, or simply an intriguing coincidence. In both yeast and paramecia, telomeres do not shorten as the cells become progressively more senescent. (In the case of paramecia, however, substantial DNA damage accumulates in the macronuclear DNA, which could in itself induce replicative senescence.) Moreover, mice have much longer telomeres than humans, but their cells do not live longer in culture.

Doubts about the role of telomeres in human replicative senescence were laid to rest in an experiment reported in the journal *Science* in early 1998. Normal human cells with the standard human replicative potential were transfected with a copy of a human gene that activates telomerase, and then grown in culture. At the time of the report, the cells receiving the telomerase-activating gene had lived half again as long as untreated cells, and showed no signs of slowing down. They were also "younger" looking in terms of cellular morphology, and the ability to adhere properly to the culture plates. The consensus at this point is that they have almost certainly escaped replicative senescence; they have likely become immortal (a not unmixed blessing, as we shall see in the next chapter).

So it is now quite certain that telomeres play a major role in the senescence of dividing cells in humans. But what is the relation of the lifespan of cells dividing in vitro to the replicative behavior of cells in vivo? It is tempting to believe that such a relationship exists: The number of cycles cells undergo in vitro is directly correlated with in vivo age, and the number of such cell cycles correlates with the maximum lifespan of a given species. There is good evidence that replicative senescence is not just something that happens to cells in vitro. Experiments have been carried out in which dividing cells were removed from one animal and their fate followed as they were passed serially from one mouse to another in vivo. These cells, when recovered and returned to culture, underwent a greatly decreased number of additional cell divisions, suggesting that winding down of replicative potential had continued in vivo.

But the overarching question really concerns the relation of replicative senescence, in vitro *or* in vivo, to the overall senescence of an organism. Replication is critical throughout life to many cells in the body: cells of the blood and immune systems, for example, or blood vessel cells. But the fact is that most cells in the body do not divide most of the time. All of the cells in adult fruit flies and roundworms, those favored models for the study of aging, are post-mitotic and never divide, yet both flies and worms age. This is one of the reasons that the claims that restoring telomerase activity in humans would lead to rejuvenation or immortality cannot be taken seriously; there is no obvious role for telomerase to play in the majority of cells in our bodies.

How do cells that are not dividing know when they are old? There is still a huge gap between molecular models based on the cell cycle, which are quite elegant and complete in terms of cell behavior in vitro, and our understanding of the aging of organisms. All available evidence suggests that the Rb-induced G_1/S block that eventually develops in cells aging in vitro also shows up in cells taken directly from very old individuals, whether dividing or not, and in dividing cells from patients with premature aging syndromes like Hutchinson-Gilford progeria and Werner's syndrome. Almost certainly the same will be true of other blocks yet undiscovered. How and why did these blocks arise in nondividing cells? And how could a G_1/S block—or any other cell cycle block—explain gray hair, wrinkled skin, heart disease, and cataracts, all of which occur in cells that are for the most part not actively dividing? We simply do not know at present.

That cell cycle control may be related in a fundamental way to the broader phenotype of senescence in the whole organism is hinted at by the identity of the gene causing Werner's syndrome. As discussed in Chapter 5, this is now known to be a DNA helicase. Helicases are one of the housekeeping genes, that is, genes expressed in each cell of the body. They are involved in unwinding the DNA in preparation either for reading genes or for repairing or replicating it. Helicases are part of the complex of proteins associated with DNA throughout the cell cycle, and interact at different stages of the cycle (particularly in S phase) with many of the proteins we have talked about in this chapter: transcription factors such as E2F and regulatory factors like the cyclins and p21. Mutations of both copies of the helicase gene in WS (for this is a recessive disease) result in an organismal phenotype that mimics perhaps one-third to one-half of the features of natural aging, including replicative senescence. This is one of the most intriguing, yet puzzling, indications of the association of cell-cycle control with senescence.

Because replicative senescence proceeds on schedule in cells removed from the body, it is clearly a cell-autonomous phenomenon; it is not directed by the brain or regulated by hormones. It proceeds according to an internal genetic program that involves some sort of counter or clock. The evidence that this program is tied to the components of the cell cycle—quite possibly telomeres—is compelling; the cell cycle is likely to be the sole basis for replicative senescence. But are the underlying causes of replicative senescence also a primary cause of senescent changes seen in other cells? Could these mechanisms trigger age-associated changes in nondividing cells similar to the changes seen in senescing fibroblasts? This is one of the key questions in the study of aging at the present time; understanding just how replicative senescence relates to aging in the entire organism will likely engage researchers for many years to come.

7

Replicative Immortality
Cancer and Aging

Although by no means restricted to the old, cancer is a disease we ordinarily associate with aging and senescence, and to a large extent this correlation is valid. For males over thirty in the United States, cancer is second only to heart attack as a cause of death in all age groups. Cancer is actually the leading disease cause of death in women between forty and sixty, but once past menopause, the incidence of cardiovascular disease increases in women, and heart attacks then exceed cancer as a cause of death in both sexes. As an age-associated idiopathic disease, cancer is very much a part of the normal process of senescence. Unquestionably, as advances in medicine and public health in this century have increased average lifespan, the proportion of deaths from cancer has increased. This is not because the frequency of cancer has increased in the population, but because other causes of death (obviously excluding cardiovascular disease) have been brought under control, unmasking an underlying association of cancer with the aging process. Cancer became a more common form of death as more people lived to an age where cancer naturally occurs.

When studied at the level of individual cells, where both cancer and replicative senescence have their origin, we see a fundamental biological connection between these two phenomena. Each can be viewed as representing a particular state of the normal eukaryotic cell cycle. In cancer, otherwise perfectly normal cells are perpetually stimulated to divide, and in addition have escaped the numerous safeguards placed throughout the cell cycle to prevent unscheduled cell division. In replicative senescence, those very same safeguards have come to dominate the mechanisms that drive the cell cycle forward, and cells can no longer respond to growth signals by entering into cell division. Whether because of this, or simply in concert with this, the senescing cell undergoes a series of changes that gradually diminish its functions, and it assumes characteristics we associate with aging.

There may seem to be as many different types of cancer as there are cells in the body, each representing almost a different disease. In practical terms, for example in the diagnosis and treatment of cancer, this is to some extent true. Yet all cancer cells have one common feature: They have lost control of the cell cycle, and thus enter into unregulated cell division. As we will see, this loss of control is caused by a combination of mutations in genes that drive the cell to divide and in the genes that suppress unscheduled cell division. Thus, every cancer originates as a disorder of the DNA itself, and all of the causes of cancer can ultimately be traced to damaged or mutated DNA.

The alterations in DNA that can lead to cancer arise in several ways. First is simple mutation, alterations in the coding sequence of DNA that may be caused by chemicals and radiation, but perhaps most often by mistakes made during DNA replication. Each time the DNA is replicated in connection with cell division, there is an opportunity for making a mistake in copying the embedded genes. The cell has extensive mechanisms for proofreading newly made DNA, and correcting any mistakes that are found, but this machinery is not completely foolproof. Mistakes may escape detection altogether or fail to trigger an appropriate repair response. Deficient DNA repair responses underlie several human clinical syndromes that show high incidences of cancer (Table 7.1). Individuals with xeroderma pigmentosum cannot repair damage to the DNA in skin cells caused by the ultraviolet radiation in

Table 7.1. *Human disorders characterized by unusually high cancer incidence*

Syndrome	Tumors commonly seen
Ataxia telangectasia	Lymphoma
Bloom's syndrome	Leukemia
Fanconi's anemia	Myeloid leukemia
Hereditary nonpolyposis colorectal cancer	Colon
Li-Fraumeni syndrome	Many different cancers seen
Xeroderma pigmentosum	Skin (including melanoma)

normal sunlight. Xeroderma sufferers have a skin cancer rate (including deadly melanomas) several thousand times greater than the general population, and a ten-fold greater rate for other types of cancer. Ataxia telangectasia is a complex disorder with a component of defective DNA repair; ataxia patients develop high levels of lymphoma. Fanconi's anemia is also characterized by a defect in the ability to repair DNA.

Physical breaks can occur in chromosomes during replication, and the open ends of DNA resulting from such breaks, lacking telomeres, can form new connections with other chromosomes, creating strange mosaic structures. On occasion, a break may occur right in the middle of a gene on one chromosome, and when that piece is joined randomly to the middle of another chromosome it may insert into the middle of a second gene. If the first gene was in an active state, that is, being "read" by the cell, it may cause the gene to which it was joined on the second chromosome to be read as well. If the gene suffering such a rude awakening happens to be a gene that triggers cellular proliferation, a tumor may result. Such translocations are common causes of leukemias. The "Philadelphia chromosome," for example, is created when a small piece of human chromosome 9 breaks off and displaces most of the long arm of chromosome 22 (Fig. 7.1), creating an abnormal hybrid chromosome. This causes the activation of a cancer-causing gene on chromosome 22. The Philadelphia chromosome is present in essentially all cases of chronic myelogenous leukemia.

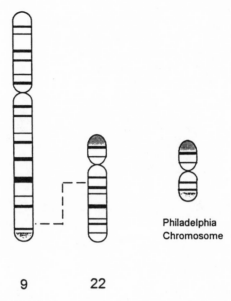

9   22

Figure 7.1. The Philadelphia chromosome found in many leukemias. The dashed line indicates the break points in chromosomes 9 and 22.

Cells are of course equipped with molecules such as p53 to detect damaged DNA, but occasionally such damage may escape detection. In the Li-Fraumeni syndrome, for instance, the p53 molecule is defective, and persons afflicted with this disorder have extraordinarily high rates of tumor development. Patients with Bloom's syndrome, which has some features of a progeria, have a high rate of chromosomal abnormalities developed during chromosomal replication. p53 is normal in these individuals, but for some reason not all of the abnormalities are detected, and the result is a high incidence of many different types of cancer. In a number of experiments with cancer cells in vitro, restoration of a functional p53 gene can revert the cancer phenotype to normal.

The Genes Associated with Cancer

One major category of genes that, when mutated, can drive normal cell division toward the development of cancer, is indicated in Figure 7.2. These genes, in their mutant form, are called oncogenes (from the Greek word for tumor, *onkos*). More than fifty oncogenes

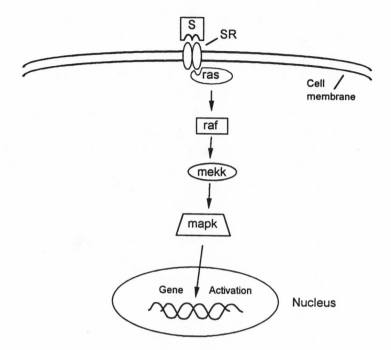

Figure 7.2. The Ras oncogene system. Cells normally begin to divide when a growth signal (S) recognizes and binds to a signal receptor (SR) in the cell's outer membrane. Molecules such as ras, located just below the membrane, sense that the receptor is occupied, and cause a chemical modification of a second molecule in the signaling pathway (raf), which activates that molecule and causes it to activate the next member of the pathway, and so on. The final step in the signaling pathway is activation of genes in the nucleus that control cell proliferation. (The names of the various components of the signaling pathway derive from short-handed notations used by the scientists who discovered them.)

have been defined in humans, and they are found in a large proportion of human tumors. All of the products of these genes are involved with receiving, transmitting, and processing growth signals. When a growth factor arrives at a cell surface, it binds to a specific receptor that recognizes that factor and no other. The receptor is itself usually a protein molecule that passes through the cell membrane. Within or immediately under the membrane, and adjacent to the receptor, are molecules that can sense when the receptor is occupied by growth factor. These molecules initiate a cascade of molecular signaling events that eventually result in a transcription factor entering the nucleus and triggering the expression of genes—such as the cyclin and Cdk genes—needed for activating the cell cycle.

This entire sequence of molecular events, from triggering the growth factor receptor through the transcription of specific genes in the DNA, is called a signaling pathway, and it is normally set in motion only by the arrival at the cell surface of the appropriate growth factor. Progression through the pathway involves sequential activation of the various components of the cascade. Each component, once activated by the preceding or "upstream" component, in turn activates the next "downstream" component, and so on until transcription is successfully initiated.

Like any other genes, the genes encoding the components of signaling pathways are subject to mutation. Some—probably most—mutations will result in production of a protein that is unable to carry out its normal function in the pathway. In this case, the cell will not be able to divide when called upon to do so, and may well die as a result, but it would not become a tumor. Some mutations may be "neutral" or "silent," causing minimal or no functional alteration in the encoded protein. A few mutations, on the other hand, will actually enhance the function of the protein, sometimes to the extent of causing inappropriate activation of the signaling pathway; it is this sort of "oncogenic" mutation that can steer a cell toward the cancerous state. For example, there are mutations in the receptor molecules themselves, which cause the receptor to behave as if it were occupied by a growth factor when it is not. None of the downstream cell cycle components are aware of this deception, and will respond just as if the cell were being bombarded by a constant stream of growth factors.

Mutations in any one of the intermediate components may also cause them to function in a constant activated or "on" state, even though all of the upstream components are at rest. The result of any one of these receptor-linked or intermediate-pathway mutations will be the activation of all proteins downstream of the mutation, eventually leading to transcription of the genes involved in entry into the cell cycle. The cell will struggle as hard as it can to respond to these never ending but false signals by dividing over and over. The Philadelphia chromosome described earlier represents just such a mutation, in this case caused by a chromosomal translocation. An oncogene called Abl is activated on chromosome 22; Abl is a member of a cell signaling pathway that triggers cellular proliferation.

It is clear from this description that oncogenes are not some alien form of disease-causing gene that has managed to infect the genome, but rather an allelic variant of a normal gene that has a specific function in the life of every normal cell. And the tumor cell itself has not become some sort of pathogenic renegade; it is just a normal cell doing its best to respond to what it perceives to be a legitimate signal to divide. Note also that for an oncogene to affect a cell, only one of the two alleles of that gene need be mutant. For example, if a cell has one normal and one mutant allele for a growth factor receptor, both normal and mutant forms of the receptor will show up in the cell's membrane. The mutant receptor in the membrane will be sufficient to drive the cell into active division, even though the unmutated receptors are well-behaved.

Oncogenes have proved very useful to viruses. Often, when a virus reproduces its DNA inside a host cell, it will clip out small pieces of the host DNA and carry them out of the cell as part of its own genome. Over evolutionary time viruses have picked up many genes in this fashion that help them in their own life cycle. Apparently some viruses have in the past infected cells with oncogenic mutations, because many of them carry around copies of human or animal oncogenes. In fact, oncogenes were first discovered as parts of viral genomes, and only later found to be slightly altered copies of normal animal genes. The viruses use these pirated oncogenes to drive the cells they infect into cell division, because dividing cells provide an expanded and more efficient environment for viral reproduction.

In many animals, infection of a particular cell by an oncogene-bearing virus may in itself be sufficient to cause cancer. In humans, where there are more effective safeguards against unscheduled cell division, virus-induced tumors are relatively rare. Certainly the cell-cycle checkpoints are a major defense against inappropriate cell division. But transformation by oncogene-bearing viruses, or mutation of cell-cycle genes into oncogenes, may drive a cell into unscheduled cell division on a fairly frequent basis, for all we know; the cells that develop into tumors in such cases may represent rare individuals that escaped detection by the immune system or other higher-level defense mechanisms.

That oncogenes alone are not generally sufficient to induce a tumor became evident when oncogenes were deliberately introduced into normal, healthy cells in culture. If the cells had potential cell divisions remaining, these might be completed, but then the cells stopped dividing. They did not become tumors. Although this seemed puzzling at the time, we now know that there are safeguards planted throughout the cell cycle to prevent unscheduled or excessive cell division. Cells are naturally resistant to fortuitous growth signals, whatever their origin. Development of full-blown cancer thus requires a simultaneous mutation in one or more of these guardians of the cell cycle, some of which were in fact originally discovered in connection with their involvement in cancer, where they were known as tumor-suppressor genes.

The first such gene to be identified in a human cancer was the Rb gene. Rb was identified as a gene for which *both copies* were either missing or seriously mutated, first in the childhood cancer retinoblastoma, and subsequently in other tumors as well. The other major cell-cycle blocker that has been identified as a tumor suppressor is p53. In fact p53 is the most commonly missing molecule associated with human cancers. (Again, both gene copies must be defective.) Its primacy in cancer defenses was made clear with the development of p53 "knock-out" mice. These mice are normal at birth and grow normally, but have an incredibly high cancer rate compared with normal mice.

While oncogenes are helpful to viruses, tumor suppressor genes are generally anathema because they block the prolific cell division needed for viruses to reproduce effectively. Many viruses have evolved proteins, such as the T antigen of SV40, to neutralize host cell tumor suppressor proteins. p53, in fact, was originally discovered as a protein bound by the proliferation-inducing T antigen; its role as a natural tumor suppressor gene was recognized only later.

The dual role played by tumor suppressor genes in cancer and in senescence is highlighted in a rather astonishing way by some very recent research into oncogene function. As just noted, when normal cells are infected with an oncogene, they do not immediately become cancerous. But in looking at this more closely, researchers found that even very young cells began "looking old" soon after infection by an oncogene called ras: The cells became larger and their shape changed in ways reminiscent of much older cells. When the contents of the cells were examined, it was found that the expression of two tumor suppressor genes—p53 and p16— had increased to very high levels, and many of the cells had arrested in G_1. Thus the cells' response to internal expression of this oncogene was to grow old before their time, to become senescent. In the case of other oncogenes, such as one called myc, the infected cells are actually instructed to commit suicide. Apparently the possibility of spontaneous mutation of oncogenes is great enough—and dangerous enough—that cells have developed means to sense when this happens, and they respond to this threat even before additional, tumor-promoting mutations have occurred. The response is similar to what happens when damaged DNA is detected during normal cell division—the cell is shunted into a state of premature senescence and in some cases driven into apoptosis. The molecular machinery for handling all of these responses is exactly the same machinery used in regulating the normal cell cycle, and in normal progression to senescence in all dividing cells.

As with most genes, a single normal allele of a tumor suppressor gene is sufficient to carry out the active function of the gene—in this case, suppression of abnormal cell division. We know this from experiments in which a single copy of an Rb gene introduced into Rb-deficient tumor cells grown in vitro was sufficient to reverse the cancer phenotype of the cell. (This strategy is the basis for several gene therapy protocols for the treatment of certain human cancers.) One faulty tumor suppressor allele would be insufficient to cause cancer; the second allele would produce more than enough of the protein that keeps cell division under control. So in the case of oncogenes, one mutant allele is sufficient to cause a problem; for tumor suppressor genes, both alleles must be mutant for tumor development. Because of this difference in a requirement for one versus two mutant alleles to cause a potential problem, so-called "hereditary cancers" never involve oncogenes. If a mutant oncogene were passed through the germ cells to a fetus, every cell in that fetus would have an active problem of excessive activation of unregulated cell division. True, for an actual tumor to develop, tumor suppressor genes would also have to be mutant. Nevertheless, the difficulty in regulating the cell cycle with a mutant signaling pathway gene distributed throughout the entire organism is bound to cause irreparable damage to a developing fetus, which would spontaneously abort. And in fact no hereditary cancer has been traced to a mutant oncogene.

On the other hand, a single faulty allele of a particular tumor suppressor gene could in fact be inherited, since the remaining "good" allele is enough to insure function. Inheritance of two faulty alleles is unlikely; it would be the equivalent of inheriting a single mutated oncogene and would cause serious problems for the developing fetus. An individual inheriting a single faulty tumor suppressor gene will not automatically develop cancer, but will have only one functional allele of that gene remaining in each and every cell of his or her body; only a single copy of the gene guards each cell against escape from cell cycle control. If at any time during the life of such an indivdual, a mutation should occur in the remaining good allele of this gene in any cell of the body, there is a very high probability that a tumor will develop from that cell. Given that there are something like a hundred trillion cells in the body, that is not at all a distant probability. Tumors of this type have been identified as resulting from inheritance of one faulty allele of either Rb or p53. What is inherited is not cancer itself, but a greatly increased likelihood that cancer might develop.

So the development of a tumor requires the mutation of several genes. There must be at least one mutation in a gene activating cell division—an oncogene—that starts the cell down the pathway toward proliferation in the absence of an appropriate signal. But there must also be a mutation in one or more of the genes whose specific purpose is to detect and suppress such events—tumor suppressor genes. Mutation of genes in either category alone, while causing problems with normal cell cycle regulation, would be unlikely to cause cancer. The need to accumulate multiple mutations in a single tumor precursor cell is one reason most cancers do not arise until relatively late in life, and why cancer is thus predominantly a disease of the elderly.

In the past few years, additional genes have been identified in humans that, when mutated, are the basis for cancers with a strong hereditary basis—certain breast and ovarian tumors (caused by the BRCA-1 and BRCA-2 genes) and hereditary colon cancers (attributed to the HNPCC-1 and -2 genes). All four of these genes behave like tumor suppressor genes, although whether or how they relate to the cell cycle is not clear at present. The BRCA-1 and -2 genes are involved in a relatively small number of strongly hereditary breast cancers (5 to 10 percent of all breast cancers) and also predispose toward ovarian cancers. Defective alleles in either of these genes can result in a 70 to 90 percent incidence of cancer in affected individuals. (A recently discovered third gene, the AT gene, may also contribute significantly to strongly hereditary breast cancer.) The HNPCC genes, which, interestingly, are involved in DNA repair, are responsible for a highly hereditary form of colon cancer called hereditary nonpolyposis colorectal cancer, which accounts for about 15 percent of colorectal cancers in the United States. An estimated one million Americans are thought to carry a disease-causing allele of one of these genes, and these individuals have a 75 percent chance of mutating a second gene and developing colon cancer in their lifetimes. There is another gene strongly predisposing to colorectal cancer called the APC gene (for adenomatous polyposis coli). It can be expected that as the Human Genome Project is brought to completion over the next ten years or so, additional genes predisposing to cancer, quite possibly involved with cell cycle regulation, will be discovered.*

Having lost the restrictions placed on them by cell-cycle regulators, cancer cells in effect gain the potential for immortality. Cell lines have been prepared from a great many human tumors, and some of these have been in continuous culture for forty years or more, giving rise to an effective biomass billions of times greater than that of the individual who begat them.** This stretch toward immortality is thwarted in vivo by the fact that the untreated tumor eventually kills its host. We saw earlier an example of transient replicative immortality expressed in the cellular descendants of the zygotes formed by normal fertilization. These cells enjoy a state of "natural" immortality that does not require genetic mutation or viral transformation. Cell lines derived

---

* The Human Genome Project is an international effort to sequence the entire human genome, thus uncovering all of the estimated 100,000 human genes. A major driving force for the Genome Project at its inception was the discovery of additional cancer-causing (or -preventing) genes. The project will likely be completed by the year 2003; unraveling the function of the genes defined may, however, require decades of additional work. For details, see William R. Clark, *The New Healers: The Promise and Problems of Molecular Medicine in the Twenty-First Century* (New York: Oxford University Press, 1997).

**Each of these cells, by the way, continues to carry a DNA "hologram" of that individual, containing all the information necessary for his or her "reassembly," as demonstrated by the recent "cloning" of a sheep from DNA from a single, fully differentiated adult sheep cell.

from these descendants, called ES cells, have been maintained in a continuous state of growth for as long as seven years, with no sign of senescence, replicative or otherwise. This is not easy to do, because the cells have a strong tendency to develop into embryos and become mortal, but it can be done. In vivo, the state represented by ES cells is thought to be very transient, lasting perhaps only until implantation of the developing embryo in the uterine wall. As far as we understand this transient immortality, it relates to a suspension, or perhaps more likely a suppression, of the normal cell-cycle controls discussed above and in the last chapter, which guard against unscheduled and unlimited cellular proliferation. It has recently been shown, for example, that ES cells have almost no Rb protein.

There is in fact little to distinguish ES cell lines and most tumor cell lines used in research today, and the underlying mechanisms of unregulated cell division appear to be the same. But in vivo, of course, as embryological development proceeds, the process of unbridled cell division is gradually brought under control, and at this point any similarity of the zygotic cells with a tumor ends. True, some cells continue to divide until the body reaches its final size and shape, months or years later. Even in the fully formed individual, many cells retain the potential to divide if called upon in an emergency—wound healing, for example. A few cells, most notably those giving rise to the various cells of the blood system, continue vigorous cell division all through life. But the story of fetal, embryological, and childhood development is one of a continual reining-in of cellular proliferation and of bringing growth processes increasingly under the most stringent regulation. This of course does not happen in cancer.

Cancer and ES cells are tied into replicative senescence through yet another aspect of the cell cycle. In the last chapter we discussed how telomeres might be involved in "counting" the number of cycles a cell has completed and shunting the cell into senescence by activating cell-cycle inhibitors such as Rb or p53. What happens with telomeres in cancer cells and ES cells, which are replicatively immortal? Remember that each time DNA replicates during S phase, telomeres lose a small portion of their total length because of the way DNA is reproduced. In more primitive eukaryotic cells where extended cell division is a normal part of a cell's life cycle, and in germ cells and a few other normally dividing cells in higher eukaryotes, telomere length is maintained by a special enzyme called telomerase, which adds additional telomeric motif units to the ends of newly replicated DNA. But telomerase is undetectable in most normal cells in the bodies of higher eukaryotes. On the other hand, it is present in high levels in both cancer cells and ES cells. It is now thought that in addition to mutations in oncogenes and tumor surpressor genes, a third type of mutation is required for a cell to become cancerous: The cell must somehow induce the reexpression of telomerase, which was among those genes shut off as embryonic differentiation proceeded. It has been proposed that the necessity to induce expression of telomerase could be the M2 barrier to cellular immortalization by viruses as well.

Another possible explanation for the appearance of telomerase in cancer cells is that some tumors may arise from developmentally primitive stem cells, which are thought to be distributed throughout most normal tissues. Stem cells represent an intermediate stage in the development of mature, fully differentiated cells, and are likely still pluripotent. This could account for the fact that many tumors look histologically undifferentiated. Stem cells are thought to be important in the local regeneration of cells and tissues, but they are extremely rare and thus difficult to find. Nonetheless, in those cases where stem cells have been identified, they appear to have a level of telomerase activity similar to germ cells or ES cells.

Telomerase has been found to be active in 90 percent or more of human tumors. This places a major constraint on the application of a recently described technique allowing scientists to introduce a telomerase gene into normal human cells. When this was done, the cells were able to grow well beyond their replicative limit; in fact at the time of this writing, they are still growing. This led some to claim that human immortality was now within reach. Certainly the cells used in these experiments have been immortalized, but of course that is also the definition of a tumor cell. The notion that telomerase activation in a living organism would increase human lifespan is a dangerous one. Reactivating telomerase in normal cells would be unlikely to convert them immediately to tumor cells, but it would remove an important barrier (M2) to unlimited proliferation in cells with altered oncogenes or tumor-suppressor genes. In that sense, cells in which telomerase had been deliberately activated would be like cells in which both copies of a tumor-suppressor gene had been lost; it could be only a single mutational event away from becoming cancerous.

The Evolutionary Origins of Cancer

For species like humans that have greatly lengthened the pre-reproductive portions of their lifespan, during which time the offspring undergoes physical, intellectual, and cultural development that enhances its reproductive success, it is important to prevent diseases like cancer from claiming the young before they in turn have a chance to reproduce. Cancer does not a priori require fifty or sixty years to develop; mice, with a lifespan of only a few years, develop cancer at about the same frequency as older humans. It may well be that mice and other short-lived animals have much less stringent safeguards against unscheduled cell division and tumor formation. From a purely biological point of view, there seems to be no reason why human beings could not develop lethal cancers in the first few years of life, and indeed a few rare (and deadly) pediatric cancers such as retinoblastoma and neuroblastoma continue to plague our offspring.

One of the ways humans have managed to defer the onset of cancer has been through the development of the powerful tumor-suppressor genes we have discussed in this and the previous chapter. These genes make it difficult to trigger unscheduled cell division, even under the influence of virally carried oncogenes. And it appears that humans also have multiple backup tumor suppressor systems, since viruses that are known to neutralize individual tumor suppressors rarely cause cancer in humans. Tumor suppressor genes would thus clearly qualify as senescence repressing genes. Regulatory genes preventing telomerase from adding telomeres to the ends of chromosomes in rapidly dividing cells may play a similar role in inhibiting the emergence of tumors from transformed cells, and thus in repressing senescence.

Telomerase itself poses an interesting dilemma in terms of inducers and repressors of senescence. From the point of view of individual cells, telomerase helps them escape from senescence, and so could be viewed as a senescence repressor. Yet from the organism's point of view, this escape from cellular senescence results in cancer, a form of organismal senescence, so telomerase looks like a senescence effector mechanism.

Cancer is one of the few instances when cellular and organismal senescence would seem to be at odds. The apparent dilemma resolves when we remember that the role of senescence in both cells and organisms is to enhance the transmission of germline DNA; the survival of organisms and the somatic cells of which they are mostly composed is always secondary to that role.

The connection between cancer and senescence, particularly replicative senescence, continues to fascinate us. Cancer is a disease unique to multicellular organisms. When cells gave up their individuality to take advantage of a communal life-style, they had to learn to live together; they had to become socialized. If any one of them chose to take a shot at immortality, it could compromise the mission of the entire organism—transmission of germline DNA to the next generation. But this is a critical consideration only before reproductive maturity; once DNA has been passed on, the need for safeguards against runaway cells is less compelling. In fact, the powerful restraints against excessive cell division that evolved to protect us against cancer when we are young are the very mechanisms that force our cells into replicative senescence when we are old. It is certainly clear from many different types of experiments that the molecular machinery in the two cases is identical. And it is also increasingly clear that replicative senescence is a feature of all senescent cells, whether or not they actively divide during most of their lifetime. Exactly how replicative senescence would become manifest as a more generalized senescence in these cells (or vice versa) is unclear at present, but remains one of the more interesting and exciting areas of aging research.

8

Caloric Restriction and Maximum Lifespan

Behind our quest for a clearer understanding of the aging process in animals doubtless lies the hope that we may somehow be able to use this information to extend our own maximum possible lifespan. For some single-cell species, maximum lifespan is to some extent a plastic quantity: It may not be defined at all in terms of calendar time, as our own lives are, but rather as a fixed number of cell divisions. In times of depleted resources, single-cell organisms can even go into a death-like state to prolong life, where they may stay for years, further complicating a precise definition of maximum lifespan. For some invertebrate species, even when maximum lifespan is defined in years or months, it can often be manipulated by relatively simple means such as changing growth temperatures. For warm-blooded mammals such as ourselves, maximum lifespan, at least in the wild, seems to be a genetically regulated property of each species, even though it may only be observable in highly artificial environments such as zoos or laboratories. Still, the fact that in organisms like roundworms and fruit flies, mutations in a single gene can result in substantial increases in maximal as well as average lifespan of 50 percent or more has led at least some researchers to ask just how predetermined maximum lifespan may be.

That maximal lifespan in warm-blooded animals—although seemingly fixed in the wild—might not be an absolutely unalterable quantity was first suggested in a believable way by experiments carried out with rats in the 1930s by the nutritionist Clive McCay at Cornell University. The type of studies McCay engaged in were stimulated at least indirectly by Buffon's suggestion in the eighteenth century that the maximal lifespan of a species could be predicted from the time it takes for members of that species to reach full physical maturity; in many mammalian species maximal lifespan is approximately five times as long as the time required for completion of body growth. McCay thus set out to determine whether postponing full physical maturity would increase maximum lifespan. To his delight and satisfaction, it seemed to do just that.

The means McCay used to retard growth in his rats was initially called dietary restriction. Although by no means the first to observe an effect of undernutrition on growth, McCay's studies were unusually well controlled, and are cited today as the true starting point for serious investigation of the interaction between nutrition and longevity. McCay allowed a portion of his rats unrestricted access to a nutritionally balanced diet. The remaining rats were fed the same diet, but restricted to about half the total amount of food. Importantly, McCay added extra vitamins and minerals to the food of those receiving a restricted diet, so that the levels of these important dietary adjuncts were the same in all groups. McCay's insistence on *under*nutrition but not *mal*nutrition set his studies apart from earlier experiments along these lines, and has been followed by all serious investigators since his time.

As expected, rats fed the restricted diet from the time they were weaned grew more slowly, and in fact never reached the size of fully fed rats, even if the restricted rats were allowed unlimited access to food later on as young adults. Nevertheless, the underfed rats appeared quite healthy, and showed no signs of physiological abnormality upon their eventual death. While alive, they had excellent coats (a sensitive sign of health problems in rodents) and later studies proved them to be quite vigorous in all exercise regimens. They did not seem to be more susceptible to infectious disease, and in fact subsequent work by McCay and others suggested that the incidence of many diseases, in particular cancer, was actually decreased in underfed rats. As McCay had hoped, the underfed rats also lived considerably longer; both the average and maximal lifespans increased by 50 to 80 percent. Researchers at the time felt that these data established quite clearly the point suggested nearly 200 years earlier by Buffon, that maximal lifespan is determined by the time required for full maturation, and if the latter is somehow retarded, the former will be extended proportionally.

McCay's observations were followed up by numerous investigators over the next two decades, who tried to identify biochemical differences between underfed and fully fed animals that could explain the effects on longevity. Dietary restriction studies were also extended to other species, both vertebrate and invertebrate and, with a few exceptions among certain invertebrates, proved to be widely true. Interest in this subject intensified in the 1970s, perhaps not coincidentally with the establishment in 1974 of the National Institute of Aging as part of the U.S. National Institutes of Health. Dozens of laboratories around the world have been intensively involved over the past two decades in diet and longevity research. As a result, our understanding of the effects of diet on longevity, and of possible underlying mechanisms, has increased considerably.

The most complete studies of the impact of dietary restriction on longevity have continued to be carried out in rats and mice. The relatively low cost of purchasing and maintaining these animals, plus the worldwide availability of genetically defined strains (which makes results easier to compare from one laboratory to another), has made them the model of choice for studying a wide range of biological questions. Moreover, years of experience in biomedical research have demonstrated that results obtained in studies with rodents can, with few modifications, provide useful information about human biology and physiology.

One of the first and most important points to emerge from the modern era of studies with rats and mice is that the single most important factor in modulating longevity is simply the total amount of calories taken in at each feeding, and the frequency of feeding. Extensive investigations of the manipulation of major food groups in the diet—

protein versus carbohydrates versus fats, alone and in various combinations—showed very clearly that complicated dietary theories concerning balances among the various food groups were not relevant to longevity. The best results were always obtained when animals were simply fed less of a well-balanced diet, as suggested by McCay over sixty years ago. As our knowledge of nutrition improved in the middle part of this century, particularly with respect to additional vitamins and trace minerals, restricted diets became much more effective in maintaining health and extending lifespan. Thus it is now more common to refer to the observed effects as due to *caloric* restriction, and not *dietary* restriction, as had been the standard practice in the several decades following McCay's first report. In most current studies of this type, total caloric intake is usually restricted to 40 to 70 percent of an unrestricted diet. Typical results are shown in Figure 8.1, which compares weight gain and survival between female rats fed an unrestricted diet and rats restricted after weaning to about 40 percent of the total

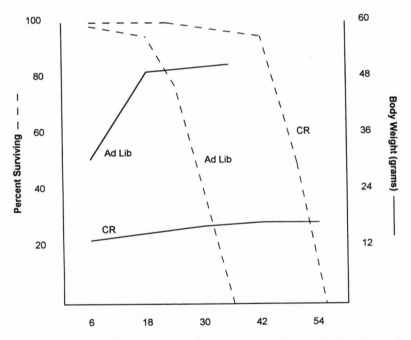

Figure 8.1. Effect of caloric restriction on weight gain and survival in female rats. In this experiment, the median survival time of the fully fed (Ad Lib) rats was 29 months; of the calorie-restricted (CR) rats, 49 months.

calories in the unrestricted diet. Calorically restricted rats weighed only a third as much as adults, compared with fully fed rats, but on average lived nearly twice as long.

The second most important fact confirmed by more recent studies is that the effect of underfeeding on longevity is not, as thought by earlier workers, due to retardation of physical growth. This is shown most clearly in studies in which caloric restriction is implemented not shortly after weaning, but only after the animals have attained full physical maturity. Although the animals may experience substantial weight loss as a result of the calorically restricted diet, their physical size does not decrease, and highly significant increases in maximal lifespan can be achieved with caloric restriction started in adults. This finding of course received a good deal of attention. No one would propose subjecting human children to caloric restriction starting in infancy, but consenting adults are another matter altogether. Thus began a fascination with the possible interactions of caloric restriction and lifespan in humans that continues to this day.

Of considerable interest are some recent studies on the effect of caloric restriction on the replicative potential of cells grown in vitro. If calorically restricted animals are, at any given calendar age, "younger" than fully fed controls, then we might expect to see this reflected in an increased potential for growth of their cells in vitro. This is indeed what is seen. Mice fed a diet containing 40 percent fewer calories than fully fed controls experienced about a 40 percent increase in maximal lifespan. When cells from a variety of tissue sites were removed for culturing in vitro, the proliferative potential of cells from the calorically restricted animals was found to be significantly greater than those taken from tissues of animals of the same calendar age given access to unlimited food. This was true at all ages except for the "oldest old"; cells at the end of life in both groups showed greatly reduced proliferative potential. However, the oldest-old calorically restricted mice were actually much older than the fully fed controls in terms of months already lived.

The impact of calorically restricted diets on virtually every aspect of the lives of experimental animals subjected to them has been examined in great detail in an attempt to understand the basis of this rather startling effect. In the following sections we examine some of the major findings of these studies.

The Effect of Caloric Restriction on Reproductive Activity

All of the studies carried out in mammals to date show a significant impact of caloric restriction on reproductive capacity. This effect is more pronounced in females than in males, most likely because of the heavier reproductive burden they carry. In one study typical for rats, females with unlimited access to food had an average onset of estrus at 40 days of age; in females fed a calorically restricted diet, the average age of first estrus was 160 days. This effect was shown to be correlated with a delayed production of reproductive hormones. However, once estrus was initiated, the rats all bore normal, healthy offspring, although litter size was generally smaller in calorically restricted females. If the level of caloric restriction is too severe, estrus may be completely suppressed, particularly in mice. However, at moderate levels of restriction, the effect appears simply to be a delay in onset of reproductive activity; calorically restricted rats are able to bear offspring well beyond the age at which control rats are reproductively senescent. In the study cited here, rats allowed unrestricted access to food were infertile by 18 months of age, whereas 80 percent of calorically restricted rats were still producing litters at this age, and a quarter of these were still reproductively active at 30 months. While on the one hand it may seem impressive that calorically restricted rats are able to reproduce at an age when control rats are reproductively senescent, in terms of their overall lifespan the reproductive period is not unusual at all, simply displaced in time in proportion to the extended lifespan of the individual rat. Nevertheless, the lifetime number of offspring produced may be somewhat less in calorically restricted animals. These results underscore the fact that it is not achievement of full body size that determines maximum lifespan, as Buffon speculated, but rather the timing of onset of reproductive activities. Because the ability to produce offspring occurs very close in time to physical maturation, it is easy to see why most scientists accepted Buffon's hypothesis.

From a biological and particularly an evolutionary point of view, all of this makes perfectly good sense. The generation of an entirely new individual (six to eight such individuals at a time for a pregnant female rat) requires enormous inputs of energy in the form of food. If a female does not have adequate food available to support her ability to produce and subsequently to nurse a litter, it is in her own interest (in terms of successful transmission of her genes to the next generation) to delay breeding activities until enough food is once again available. This reluctance to breed would be expected in terms of many of the evolutionary models discussed in Chapter 3, particularly the "disposable soma" model of Kirkwood and associates, which predicts that animals will not invest scarce resources in unsuccessful reproductive activities that might threaten their existence. Given the general thesis that initiation of senescence is deferred in animals until they initiate reproduction, the delay in reproductive activities caused by caloric restriction would be expected to lengthen maximal lifespan. Because it is females that carry the major resource-requiring burden in reproduction, it makes sense that the life-extending effects of caloric restriction are seen most clearly in that sex.

Sexual development in rats, as in humans, is regulated by hormones produced in the hypothalamus and pituitary gland. It is perhaps not surprising that the effects of underfeeding on breeding behavior are found to be accompanied by a perturbation of the associated hormonal patterns. Exactly how or why caloric restriction could affect hormonal patterns in the brain is unclear, but the genes for sex hormones are good candidates for senescence regulator genes. Altered hormone patterns, and the accompanying alterations in reproductive behavior (including earlier reproductive senescence), return to normal in calorically restricted rats returned to a normal diet.

Effects of Caloric Restriction on Disease

The diseases that characterize the later stages of life in all warm-blooded animals are largely idiopathic, that is, of self origin—cardiovascular disease, cancer, and stroke, for example—but many such diseases also render the individual more susceptible to accidental death. Any decline from the physical peak of the pre-reproductive years may result in failure to escape from a predator or compete for food, or in an increased susceptibility to "accidental" diseases caused by infectious microorganisms. For a variety of reasons, the most extensively studied age-associated idiopathic disease in animals is cancer. Over the past fifty years numerous studies in rodents have demonstrated conclusively that even moderate caloric restriction has a profound inhibitory effect on the development of tumors. Both the age of onset and the total incidence of virtually every known tumor are altered in calorically restricted animals. Moreover, animals on restricted diets survived on average half again as long with their tumors, once they developed, compared with fully fed controls.

A possible basis for the effect of caloric restriction on the development of chemically induced tumors was recently reported in the journal *Cancer Research*. Mice were fed a carcinogen known to cause bladder cancer. This tumor usually shows up at multiple sites in the bladder, and is highly invasive in the surrounding tissues. Some of the treated mice were given unlimited access to food, and some were put on a calorically restricted diet. The fully fed mice all developed multiple, highly invasive tumors in their bladders. Only a few of the calorically restricted mice developed tumors; these were single tumors, and they did not invade surrounding tissues. The researchers noted that a protein called IGF-1, which is known to make certain human tumors resistant to treatment, was considerably depressed in the calorically restricted mice. To see whether the reduced levels of IGF-1 might be responsible for the reduced cancer incidence, an additional batch of calorically restricted mice was injected with the tumor-inducing agent, and at the same time with purified IGF-1 protein. Mice receiving IGF-1 injections were as susceptible to the induced bladder cancer as fully fed mice. How caloric restriction affects IGF-1 production is unknown, but is currently under investigation. It is assumed, although not yet proved, that lowered levels of IGF-1 are also responsible for the decreased level of spontaneous cancers seen in calorically restricted mice. It will also be of great interest, of course, to determine just how lowered levels of IGF-1 make mice more resistant to tumor development.

Although other diseases have not been as intensively studied as cancer, the same pattern appears to hold true. The onset of spontaneous lung and kidney disease, the extent of bone and muscle degeneration, and the incidence of vascular diseases are all greatly retarded in rats maintained on a restricted diet, as is the frequency and severity of disorders such as ulcers, hypertension, and cataracts. In one study using a strain of rats genetically predisposed to end-stage kidney disease, renal degeneration was found in 56 of 80 control rats dying between 18 and 24 months, but in none of the calorically restricted rats, all of whom died between 18 and 48 months. Reflecting the effect of caloric restriction on extension of lifespan, a significant delay or reduction of disease was achieved with both infant- and adult-onset caloric restriction.

As with the impact of caloric restriction on reproductive behavior, the underlying mechanisms behind retardation of disease are in most cases not immediately obvious. For many years after McCay's initial report, biochemists eagerly analyzed the inner workings of calorically restricted animals. This was, after all, the great age of biochemistry (1940–70), and all of the advances made in that field were applied in an attempt to understand and explain the effect of limiting caloric intake. Virtually every enzyme system and metabolic pathway was dissected and examined in great detail, but it must be admitted that the majority of these studies provided only minimal information that would help us understand how caloric restriction could delay breeding, extend lifespan, and retard disease. All of the metabolic and physiological systems examined in calorically restricted animals were, at any given age, equivalent to those of much younger animals fed an unrestricted diet. The most likely biological explanation for accelerated aging in fully fed animals at present centers on something called oxidative stress, which will be explored in detail in the next chapter.

The Effect of Caloric Restriction on the Immune System

Caloric restriction delays the normal, age-associated degeneration of almost all of the body's physiological systems, which is the basis for the observed extension of maximal lifespan in calorically restricted animals. The role of the immune system in normal aging has itself been extensively investigated, and there have been suggestions that the impact of caloric restriction on immune function may be the key to understanding the impact of caloric restriction on longevity. What happens in the immune system in fully fed versus calorically restricted animals is likely typical of most of the body's major systems, so let's look at some of these changes in detail.

Immune function ordinarily declines substantially with age after onset of reproductive maturity. Although this decline is unlikely to be a primary cause of aging per se, a decrease in the ability to combat infectious disease is unquestionably a major cause of accidental morbidity and mortality in older animals. The crippling effects of autoimmune diseases in older animals would negatively affect their ability to seek out and to compete for food, and to escape from predators. The immune system is also an important defense against cancer, a disease that would clearly affect performance in the wild, even before it led to death of the animal itself. Thus the impact of caloric restriction on age-associated immune function in animals has been a major target for investigation by several laboratories in the past two decades.

There are a number of immune parameters that change with age, and that are presumed to underlie diminished immune capacity. One of the most prominent age-associated changes occurs in the thymus. The thymus is an organ lying just above the heart, and it is vitally involved in the production of one of the body's most important defenses against disease, the white blood cells called T cells. At about the time that reproductive activities begin, the thymus begins gradually to shrink in size, and slows its production of T cells. In very old animals (including humans) the thymus is essentially nonexistent. The detailed cellular makeup of the thymus also changes with age, and the portion of the thymus most involved in new T-cell generation (the cortex) is the most sensitive to age-related changes. In calorically restricted mice, although the thymus (like other organs in the body) is somewhat smaller than normal, the age-related shrinkage and degeneration of the cortex is greatly retarded; at any given age, the cortex of a thymus from a calorically restricted mouse looks very much like the cortical thymus in a much younger animal.

A study of the white blood cells in the circulation of calorically restricted mice has revealed a much longer period of robust T-cell function than in fully fed controls. As animals age, their T cells become increasingly less responsive to signals that ordinarily induce them to proliferate and help fight infection. These poorly responsive T cells accumulate in older animals, where they eventually come to predominate. Together with slower production of new T cells from the thymus, this results in markedly reduced T-cell responses to challenge by invading germs. Although the overall number of white cells is reduced in calorically restricted mice, the proportion of young, healthy T cells is much higher than in the controls, especially the critical subset of T cells called "helper T cells," also known as CD4 T cells.

Helper T cells play several key roles in immune responsiveness

(Fig. 8.2). They provide important chemical amplifiers to other white blood cells called B cells, which make the antibody used to clear microbes from the bloodstream, and to so-called "killer" T cells, which destroy virally infected self cells. (Helper T cells are also the cells selectively destroyed in AIDS.) In calorically restricted animals, the proportion of healthy, responsive helper T cells in the overall population is considerably increased. As a result, the T-cell responses of calorically restricted animals to a variety of challenges are unusually robust, and correspond at any given age to responses seen in much younger animals. Studies of another white cell type called the "natural killer" (NK) cell, thought to be important in defenses against tumors, showed that these cells were also unusually strong in older calorically restricted animals. NK-cell function in lymphoid tissues such as the spleen and lymph nodes also normally declines with age; this decline was markedly delayed in animals on a calorically restricted diet.

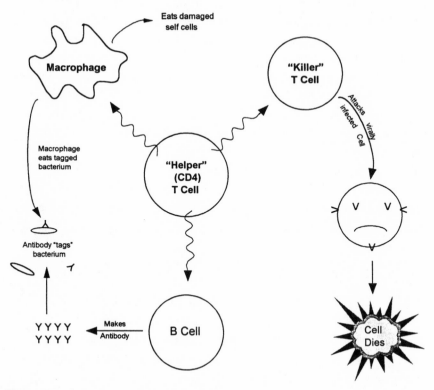

Figure 8.2. Cellular interactions in the immune response.

Other age-associated changes in the immune system are also ame-
liorated by controlled underfeeding. One of the best animal models for
autoimmunity is the NZB/W mouse, which spontaneously develops a
broad-spectrum, lupus-like disease as it approaches sexual maturity.
Systemic lupus erythematosis is one of the most common chronic,
debilitating autoimmune diseases in humans, affecting predominantly
(but not exclusively) women. When NZB/W mice were placed on a
calorically restricted diet after weaning, the onset of symptoms of this
disease was greatly delayed, and in many cases completely prevented.
Mice placed on a restricted diet after onset of their disease also showed
less severe disease complications, including the kidney damage that is
a concomitant of almost all autoimmune diseases. They became more
active and lived significantly longer than the fully fed controls.

So caloric restriction does indeed have a profound effect on the
immune system, resulting in a younger, healthier immune system, better able to fight infectious disease and cancer and to avoid autoimmune
problems. All of the effects observed would obviously be advantageous
for average lifespan, and could conceivably contribute to maximum
lifespan as well. But the same is probably true of increased performance
by most of the body's major physiological systems, all of which are also
seemingly rejuvenated by a caloric restriction regimen. There is no reason to believe that improved immune function is any more important
for longevity than improved kidney, lung, or heart function. It seems
very likely that these improved performances are all a reflection of
some more fundamental biological alteration, resulting in better survival and performance of the cells of which these various systems are
composed. The opposite side of the coin, of course, is that unrestricted
feeding may be accelerating the aging process through these same fundamental mechanisms.

Caloric Restriction in Higher Primates and Humans

Intensive studies carried out over nearly two decades in
species as wide ranging as roundworms, fruit flies, rats, and mice, have
been remarkably consistent in showing that caloric restriction increases
both average and maximal lifespan. These species were selected for
study in part because they have lifespans sufficiently short that an
impact of diet could be measured with reasonable amounts of experi-

mental time and effort. The question that is of course at the back of everyone's mind is whether we could expect to see the same impact of a calorically restricted, nutritionally balanced diet on lifespan in humans, particularly if restriction could be initiated in adults.

To gain further insight into this possibility, several studies have been initiated with primates whose overall physiology and genetic constitution are very close to humans. One such study has been organized through the National Institutes of Health's Primate Unit in Poolesville, Maryland. Beginning in April 1987, thirty rhesus monkeys in three age groups (juveniles, 7–12 months of age; adolescents, 3–5 years of age; and old, 18–25 years of age) were entered into the study. The first two groups were each divided into two subgroups, one of which received a normal, full diet, and one of which received 30 percent fewer calories overall, with a vitamin and mineral supplement to bring them up to par nutritionally with the fully fed subgroup.

Six years into the study, monkeys kept on a calorically restricted diet weighed significantly less than fully fed controls, but were extremely healthy and performed physically as well as the controls. One of the more intriguing findings to date is that calorically restricted monkeys, like many (but not all) of the calorically restricted animals in previous studies, have a core body temperature that is slightly but significantly lower than that seen in fully-fed controls. The difference in this case was about half a degree centigrade during the day, and one degree centigrade during sleep. This would represent a considerable reduction in calories burned for purposes of maintaining body temperature. Although it will likely be twenty years or more before we will know whether lifespan has been increased in these monkeys, all indications to date are that the early responses to caloric restriction in these animals are comparable to the early responses to caloric restriction seen in other animals where a significantly increased maximum lifespan was achieved. In another study with rhesus monkeys, measuring energy used across a twenty-four-hour day, it was found that calorically restricted monkeys expended much less energy at night than did fully fed animals, which is consistent with the findings on body temperature.

In a recently initiated study using a strain of monkeys that has a high incidence of spontaneous atherosclerosis and heart disease, a diet was created that contained 30 percent fewer calories, but had the same level of cholesterol as the animals' normal diet. After one year, monkeys fed the calorically restricted diet showed substantial weight loss and a marked reduction in fat (particularly abdominal fat). They also showed an enhanced response to insulin. The results of this study, as they unfold, will be of particular interest because they may point to what we could expect the impact of caloric restriction to be on one of the most important human senescence-related diseases, namely, cardiovascular disease.

An important question to ask about caloric restriction is what impact it may have on the quality of life. This is uniquely a human question, entirely subjective, and not one that can be answered directly from animal studies. Although all of the primates kept on restricted diets so far are certainly healthy, we cannot ask them how they feel about it. Would humans subjected to a calorically restricted diet be constantly hungry, spending all of their free time and energy thinking about food, and how to get it? Would we be constantly agitated and irritable because we're chronically hungry? To achieve an extended lifespan, would we have to reduce our total energy expenditure, foregoing many of the energy-expensive activities that enrich our lives? These are complex and important questions to which we may never really know the answers.

An experimental analysis of the effects of caloric restriction on maximum lifespan per se in humans is probably not practical. Maintaining large numbers of people under rigidly controlled conditions of caloric intake throughout their entire lives, no matter how committed and enthusiastic they may be initially, simply cannot be done. But shorter trials to look at the early responses to caloric restriction may be revealing. In September 1991, four men and four women of excellent initial health voluntarily entered into Biosphere 2, where they remained for a period of two years. Biosphere 2 is a three-acre compound near Tucson, Arizona, built originally to test the feasibility of biologically self-sufficient human living units that might be involved in extraterrestrial exploration. (The complex was named Biosphere 2 in recognition of the earth itself as Biosphere 1.) One of the objectives was to raise all required food internally, to recycle solid, liquid, and gaseous waste products, and generally to remain independent of outside support (other than energy from the sun).

Although not part of the original plan for living in the Biosphere, the "Biospherians" adopted what was in effect a calorically restricted diet, which was largely vegetarian, supplemented by small amounts of fish and animal meat. Three meals a day were served, and all food served was consumed. The average total calories consumed per day was about 1800; fat was kept to a maximum of 30 percent of the total calories consumed, and care was taken to keep a proper balance of major food groups. One of the members of the group, Dr. Roy Walford, was a physician who had also been a pioneer in the animal studies defining the effect of caloric restriction on longevity and on immune function. He himself had been experimenting with a calorically restricted diet for some years prior to Biosphere 2. Dr. Walford monitored a number of physiological parameters in the Biospherians that might be expected to be affected by a restricted diet. After just six months on the Biosphere diet, weight losses ranged from 10 to 15 percent. Average blood pressures dropped 20 percent, cholesterol levels dropped by 35 percent, and serum lipids by 31 percent. While it would be risky to attribute these changes entirely to diet, it must be admitted that these changes parallel closely those seen in previous studies of animals, particularly higher primates, maintained on calorically restricted diets.

Continuance of the physiological studies on the Biospherians eventually had to be suspended because of problems in maintaining the proper balance of gases in the enclosed atmosphere, and further scientific evaluation of the effect of caloric restriction on human parameters that might be related to aging was abandoned. But a related study carried out in Holland supports the findings of Biosphere 2. In the Dutch study, twenty-four healthy male volunteers, thirty-five to fifty years of age, were entered into a twelve-week regimen in which they lived at home and continued their normal daily routines, but ate all of their meals under supervision of the researchers. Their daily caloric intake was reduced by 20 percent, largely through reductions of fat and sugar, and vitamin and mineral supplements were given where deemed appropriate. Those placed on a restricted diet lost 10 percent of their body weight, and experienced decreases in serum cholesterol and in blood pressure. These individuals performed as well on physical and mental tests as fully fed controls.

Based on these preliminary human studies, the initial results with higher primates, and the clear demonstration in rodents and other animals that adult-onset caloric restriction can be effective in increasing lifespan, it seems reasonable to imagine that similar effects could be achieved in humans. Accordingly, a group of interested scientists and physicians (including Dr. Walford) has drafted a plan for an open-living study in humans of the effects of caloric restriction on human lifespan. The objective of such a study obviously cannot be to determine an effect on maximal longevity per se, since that would take hundreds of years and involve impossible logistical problems. Rather, the study would focus on those parameters known from animal studies most likely to have an impact on maximum lifespan. The diet would be similar to those described above, and would initially involve individuals in the twenty-five- to thirty- and fifty-five- to sixty-year-old age ranges. Weekly recordings of dietary consumption and measurements of health statistics would be used to monitor progress through the program. Individuals would spend up to two years in the program. When such a study might actually get under way is uncertain at present.

What Does It All Mean?

The data showing that caloric restriction can improve health and increase lifespan in animals is overwhelmingly convincing. Perhaps, though, we should phrase this statement differently. Animals in the wild are probably chronically restricted calorically. Very few animals living naturally would have the luxury of the unrestricted feeding patterns enjoyed by most laboratory animals, free of the threat of predators, with no need to compete for scarce resources. So it may be that what the data are telling us is not that caloric restriction can make us healthier and live longer, but that over-eating and minimal exercise can decrease our quality of life and make us die sooner. We do not really know what an appropriate calorically restricted diet for humans would be, other than that it should be nutritionally balanced. But it is abundantly clear that human beings can subsist on many fewer calories than is typical in most industrialized countries; simply look at diets in less-developed countries. People on such involuntarily calorically restricted diets often do not fare well in terms of health and lifespan, but that is almost certainly due to improper overall nutrition and the suboptimal general medical care they receive compared with individuals in wealthier countries, not the number of calories they consume.

Remember that the keynote in all caloric restriction studies in animals has been *under*nutrition but not *mal*nutrition. That we live as long as we do in industrialized societies is likely because of vastly improved public health and medical care, and not to our calorie-rich diets. The implications are that the apparent maximal lifespan for human beings of between 110 and 120 years that we think we see at the present time may not be the true human limit after all. At the very least, the data from all of the studies so far suggest that extended average lifespans, and improved quality of life, are readily within reach for humans as well as other animals through caloric restriction. It may be as simple as returning our forks to the side of our plates a few minutes earlier each time we eat.

9

With Every Breath We Take

Oxidative Stress and Cellular Senescence

It is now beyond question that caloric restriction can have a profound impact on both average and maximal lifespan. But how are we to explain this effect, which can be observed in virtually every species? We could imagine that animals reared on a calorically restricted diet are simply healthier, and as a result live longer. That could perhaps explain the increase in average lifespan, but it is not at all obvious how such factors could affect maximum lifespan, which, to the extent that it is genetically determined, would not be expected under normal conditions to vary on anything less than an evolutionary time scale.

If the conclusion stated at the end of the last chapter is true, that what the caloric restriction experiments are telling us is that overfeeding may prevent us from realizing our true maximum lifespan, then it may well be that in these experiments we are touching on something very fundamental to the aging proccess. We have said before that in order to understand aging, we must search for basic senescence mechanisms that are common to all cells, mechanisms that when set in motion could explain the enormous range of phenotypes associated with the aging process. We imagine such mechanisms must involve something extremely fundamental to life—more fundamental, even, than eating. Perhaps as fundamental as the air we breathe.

Oxygen: The Precious Poison

We are all aware of how dependent we are on oxygen. It is the most crucial element in every breath we take, the stuff upon which our very life depends. Deprivation of oxygen for even a few minutes, for example, in connection with a heart attack or interference with breathing, can lead to fatal consequences for heavily oxygen-dependent parts of the body such as the brain. But we are perhaps less aware of how incredibly toxic oxygen can be. When life first appeared on earth some three to four billion years ago, the atmosphere was largely devoid of gaseous oxygen. Early bacterial life forms, like the anaerobic bacteria that still survive today, did not use oxygen in the process of breaking down food to generate energy. The gradual increase in the concentration of oxygen in the atmosphere that occurred around two billion years ago (caused by hydrogen-hungry, water-splitting photosynthetic cyanobacteria, some of which would later become the oxygen-generating parts of plants) was an evolutionary challenge of major proportions. Before the cyanobacteria, oxygen was at best a trace element in the atmosphere; it would eventually reach current levels of about 20 percent. Oxygen is a deadly, corrosive gas, causing iron to crumble into rust and wreak havoc with nearly all of the organic molecules on which life is based. The release of oxygen into the atmosphere by cyanobacteria forced all other life forms on earth to develop specializations to protect themselves against oxidative degradation. There was no choice; those that failed to do so simply did not survive.

As atmospheric oxygen began to mount, the evolutionary descendants of the bacteria—the eukaryotic *Protista*—were beginning to expand rapidly into a wide range of ecological niches. Like bacteria, the protists were still single-cell organisms, but they became very large; eventually they became multicellular and evolved into the plants and animals that dominate the earth today. The protists were also faced with the challenge of surviving in an increasingly toxic, oxygen-filled environment. One of the means they developed for dealing with oxygen involved a process called endosymbiosis. Certain bacteria had already developed quite good defenses against oxygen, including not just the means to neutralize it, but the ability to use it to produce energy. The ability to generate large amounts of energy very quickly was a major advantage of oxygen over other energy-generating systems that had been tried, and led to the rapid adoption of the oxygen pathway in spite of its high toxicity. Some of the oxygen-using bacteria apparently found the interiors of the larger, more advanced protists a reasonable place to live and raise a family; they became symbiotic intracellular parasites. The protists could have simply digested these intruders for food; instead, they converted them into permanent parts of the protist cell and put them to work dealing with the protists' own oxygen toxicity problem. This may not have been what the bacteria had in mind when they came aboard, but the experiment turned out to be so successful that eventually all eukaryotic cells acquired similar intracellular parasites.

Ultimately, the intracellular bacteria lost their individual identities altogether and became a working part of the protist cell. We find these bacterial "living fossils" in our own cells to this day: They became the mitochondria, the highly specialized, oxygen-consuming, energy-producing organelles found today in every eukaryotic animal cell. It is rather easy now to see their prokaryotic origins: Only the mitochondria, of all the organelles inside a cell, have their own DNA, showing their independent biological origin. This DNA is single-stranded and usually circular, and contains genes that are distinctly prokaryotic rather than eukaryotic in structure. But when this radical evolutionary origin for mitochondria was first proposed by Lynn Margulis in the early 1970s, nearly a decade passed before it was widely accepted. It is possible that other organelles within the eukaryotic cell have a similar origin, but the traces are not so clear.

The mitochondria are the site within each cell where oxygen is combined with enzymatically degraded food products to produce energy. The molecular form of the energy produced in the mitochondria is something called adenosine triphosphate (ATP). Greater than 90 percent of the oxygen consumed by an average animal cell is burned in the mitochondria to produce ATP. The basic chemical reaction that occurs during ATP generation is the opposite of that taking place in the oxygen-producing cyanobacteria (and in all plants): The mitochondria combine oxygen with hydrogen to form water, and use the energy thus released to form ATP.

Oxygen in its gaseous form (O_2) and as a component of water (H_2O) is fairly stable, but during the transformation from O_2 to H_2O in the cell a number of potentially reactive oxygen intermediates are generated (Fig. 9.1). Although the vast majority of the intermediates generated are processed right on through to the water stage during energy generation, inevitably a few escape from the reaction site; this "leakage" has been estimated to be several percent of the total oxygen processed by the cell. It is these escaped intermediate forms, called reactive oxygen species (which we will refer to simply as oxygen radicals), that are responsible for the oxygen toxicity that is so deadly to other components of the cell. Oxygen radicals produced in the mitochondria include the superoxide anion, hydrogen peroxide, and hydroxyl "free radicals," the latter of which in particular can attack and seriously damage a wide range of cellular molecules, including membrane lipids, cellular proteins, and, perhaps most important, DNA.

Oxygen radicals include some of the most potent DNA mutagens known. The mitochondria themselves are one of the primary victims of this form of "biological rusting," perhaps because of their proximity to these metabolically generated toxic wastes. Eukaryotes protect their DNA from all sorts of assaults by wrapping it in protective proteins called histones. As in their prokaryotic predecessors, the DNA of mitochondria is not protected by histones, and is thus more susceptible to direct oxidative attack. Damage to mitochondria will of course affect energy production within cells, compromising almost every function critical to their health. And mitochondrial damage is self-compounding; when damaged, mitochondria become even more leaky,

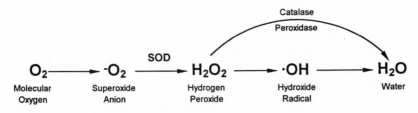

Figure 9.1. Generation of reactive oxygen species during metabolism of oxygen.

spilling more oxygen radicals into their immediate vicinity. This mito-chondrial degradation is thought to be a major contributor to cellular senescence.

Although mitochondria are clearly the major source of oxygen radicals within the cell, there are several other intracellular sources of oxidative by-products. Oxygen diffuses into cells from the surrounding extracellular fluids, and is quickly sequestered within the mitochondria. However, while molecular oxygen (O_2) is passing through the cytoplasm on its way to the mitochondria, it can undergo spontaneous degradation, particularly if it comes in contact with molecules containing iron or copper, which catalyze the generation of oxygen radicals, particularly peroxides. Normally iron and copper are kept tightly bound to special chaperone proteins like ferritin or ceruloplasmin, but in some situations—prematurely born babies, for example—free forms of iron or copper may be available to catalyze the breakdown of oxygen. There is also another cellular organelle called the peroxisome, where excess fats and other molecules are degraded using oxygen. Ridding cells of such molecules is essential to their survival, but peroxisomes can be a significant source of reactive oxygen species under certain dietary conditions. Another intracellular radical-generating site is the cytochrome P450 system of the liver, which has a special mechanism for the oxidative destruction of external toxins that manage to breach the cell's outer membrane. Finally, incidental cosmic radiation impinging on a cell can result in generation of oxygen radicals; this is probably the major cause of skin degeneration in people exposed to excessive sunlight. With the exception of the latter effect, however, all of these extramitochondrial sources ordinarily do not account for more than 10 percent of the oxygen radicals generated.

One of the more common sources of reactive oxygen species in the body as a whole is from cells that use the destructive power of these molecules as a natural defense against microbial invasion. Phagocytes (literally, "eaters of cells") such as macrophages and neutrophils purposely generate high levels of oxygen radicals, which they store in tightly sealed intracellular compartments. When phagocytes engulf bacteria or other microbes during the course of an infection, they deliver them to these internal radical-containing compartments, where they are very efficiently destroyed. Unfortunately, after several rounds of microbial feeding, the phagocytes die and release their contents into the surrounding tissues. Oxygen radicals released in this fashion can be taken up by adjacent cells, and once inside they cause the same sort of damage as radicals produced internally. For infections that are rapidly and efficiently cleared, the damage caused by phagocytic oxygen radical spillage is usually negligible. But in the case of prolonged infections, a chronic inflammatory state may develop, and the repeated engorging and death of phagocytes can cause serious oxidative damage to nearby healthy cells. This is also the major source of damage in chronic inflammatory autoimmune reactions such as rheumatoid arthritis, and can lead to serious tissue loss. Particularly in older individuals in whom oxidative damage repair processes may be less efficient, the cumulative effects of oxygen radicals can be serious indeed.

The damage done by reactive oxygen molecules to the biological molecules needed to operate living cells can be enormous. No molecular species is immune. Oxygen radicals can attack and deform protein molecules, disrupting structural complexes and inhibiting important enzymatic functions. Protein degradation products frequently show up in the body fluids of elderly persons or of patients with chronic infections or chronic inflammatory diseases such as arthritis. Various lipid oxidation products show up in pigment granules called lipofuscin that clog the cells of older individuals, and are a major component of atherosclerotic plaques. Oxygen radicals also attack the individual nucleotide bases that make up both nuclear and mitochondrial DNA.

To protect themselves from external as well as internal oxidative damage, eukaryotic cells have developed a number of defenses that either neutralize oxygen radicals before they cause serious harm or quickly repair any damage they may do. Oxygen circulating throughout the body is kept tightly bound to hemoglobin, which prevents it from damaging other components of blood or attacking and destroying the blood vessels themselves. Once oxygen radicals have been produced inside a cell, there are enzymes dedicated to destroying or otherwise neutralizing reactive oxygen species that may stray from the reaction site. Cytoplasmic superoxide dismutase converts the superoxide anion to hydrogen peroxide, which can then be disposed of by protective enzymes such as catalase and the various peroxidases (Fig. 9.1). There are also mechanisms for repairing or getting rid of damaged lipids and proteins. But of most concern in terms of senescence is what happens to DNA. The damage to DNA caused by oxygen radicals is essentially the same as that caused by radiation; as we know, unrepaired DNA damage in cycling cells can result in the induction of p53 and arrest of the cell cycle. The number of "hits" on the DNA in a single cell by oxygen radicals has been estimated to be on the order of tens of thousands per day.

DNA repair in higher animals is not well understood, and most of what we know about this process has been learned from studying bacteria and other single-cell organisms. Single-cell organisms are particularly vulnerable. They are often exposed to very high levels of light and other cosmic radiation, and they are more directly exposed to environmental chemicals that can damage DNA. Thus they tend to have highly efficient DNA repair systems. Interestingly, the DNA damage caused by reactive oxygen molecules or radiation is not itself a significant cause of mutations to genes. Rather, it is mistakes made during the DNA repair process that most often induces mutations. The same appears likely to be true in animal cells; as far as can be determined, DNA repair in higher animals generally conforms to what has been learned by studying lower organisms.

The most common repair mechanism, employed when hydroxyl radicals attack individual DNA bases, is something called nucleotide excision repair. A large number of proteins are involved in this procedure. Some detect that a base mismatch has occurred between opposing strands of DNA, usually because the double helix at mismatched sites is physically distorted. Separate sets of proteins are then involved in cutting out the mismatched nucleotide, replacing it with the correct one, and connecting the new nucleotide to its neighbors on either side. But many aspects of the repair process are still not understood. For example, at the site of a mismatch, how does the repair system know which of the two opposing nucleotides is the good one, and which the bad? We simply do not know. Nevertheless, there is good experimental evidence that DNA repair, including repair of telomeric DNA, declines with age and could thus contribute to cellular senescence through induction of the p53 pathway.

The Oxidative Stress Hypothesis of Aging

All of these observations led a number of scientists to formulate the oxidative stress hypothesis of aging, wherein senescence at the cellular level is proposed to result from cumulative damage caused by toxic oxygen intermediates. In the context of this hypothesis, aging is seen as the sum of unrepaired oxidative injuries at the cellular level, triggering idiopathic disease, which renders an individual more susceptible to accidental death and which may in itself be fatal (e.g., cancer or cardiovascular disease). The net result in terms of damage over time will reflect a balance between the rate of production of oxygen radicals and the effectiveness of prevention or repair of the cellular damage they cause, particularly to DNA. Cancer, as one example, is a major element of post-reproductive senescence in both long- and short-lived animals, and unrepaired damage to DNA is known to be a major cause of cancer.

The oxidative stress hypothesis could also help explain differences we see in maximal lifespan across different species. The early entrance into the senescent state that we see in short-lived organisms would represent a tip in the balance between damage and repair toward the accumulation of cellular damage early in life. Longer-lived species would either generate less oxidative damage to begin with or have

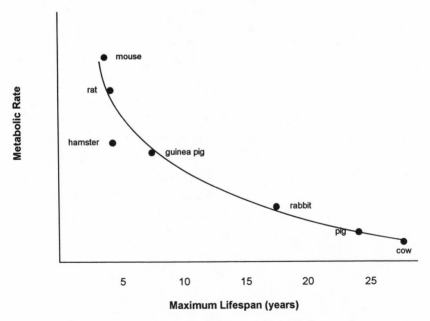

Figure 9.2. The correlation of maximum lifespan with metabolic rate.

more effective prevention or repair mechanisms in place for a longer period of time.

Supportive evidence for the oxidative stress hypothesis comes from a number of directions. One piece of indirect evidence is the correlation of maximum lifespan with overall metabolic rate (Fig. 9.2). Higher metabolic rates mean more energy produced per unit time, which will result in a greater rate of oxygen radical production, and animals with racier metabolisms do tend to have shorter average and maximal lifespans. This is likely exacerbated by the fact that most of them do not have enhanced repair systems in place to balance the oxidative damage resulting from a heavier oxygen radical burden. Longer-lived animals generally have lower steady-state levels of radicals in their cells, at least prior to sexual maturation, and this appears to be due mostly to higher levels of both antioxidants and damage repair mechanisms. This changes with age.

There is good evidence that lifespan, particularly in primates, correlates very well with the level of circulating antioxidants. Studies in many different laboratories have shown that cells taken from older members of longer-lived species, including humans, are more susceptible to oxidative damage in vitro than are younger cells. They seem less able to neutralize oxygen radicals to begin with, and are also slower to repair radical- or radiation-induced DNA damage. Mitochondria from older cells have been shown to "leak" more oxygen radicals per unit of oxygen consumed. The overall trend of these studies strongly suggests an increasing accumulation of oxidative damage with age in longer-lived animals.

Studies with human fibroblasts have been particularly informative. The number of doublings fibroblasts grown in vitro can undergo is strongly influenced by the concentration of oxygen to which they are exposed. Human cells are normally grown in vitro in the presence of 20 percent oxygen, for no other reason than that is the concentration of oxygen found in the atmosphere, and this was the condition adopted by those who developed the techniques for cell culture early in this century. This has been the oxygen concentration used to analyze the proliferative capacity of human fibroblasts of various ages in the vast majority of studies carried out to date.

But in fact, oxygen tension within the body itself is much less than

20 percent, more on the order of 3 percent. When fibroblasts were cultured in vitro under 3 percent oxygen, the number of doublings at any given age increased by 50 percent or more. In a different study, the oxygen concentration was doubled to 40 percent, and the number of cell doublings was greatly reduced. The fibroblasts cultured under this unusually high oxygen concentration quickly accumulated the characteristics of senescent cells, including gross enlargement and the accumulation of lipofuschin granules in their cytoplasm. Interestingly, the DNA in these cells showed greatly shortened telomeres, confirming once again the close correlation of telomere length and senescent status in dividing cells.

The toxic effect of higher concentrations of oxygen itself, or of preformed oxygen radicals, can be offset if antioxidants are added to the culture medium. In one study, radicals such as superoxide anion and hydrogen peroxide were tested against human fibroblasts of various ages growing in a dish. Older fibroblasts had a much more difficult time dealing with these challenges, apparently because of reduced levels of intracellular antioxidants. In another study, it was shown that preformed oxygen radicals added to the culture medium of young human fibroblasts decreased the number of cell doublings by 35 percent compared with untreated controls. These cells acquired all of the features of senescent cells, in terms of both their cellular metabolism and their external morphology. Thus not only do older human cells grown in culture show signs of considerable oxidative damage and an impaired ability to repair such damage with increasing age, but younger cells can be brought to a stage of accelerated senescence by exposure to oxidative byproducts. But when antioxidants were added simultaneously to the cultures, all of these effects were completely reversed.

The importance of natural antioxidants to aging in vivo was borne out in a set of experiments carried out at the University of Texas, in which extra copies of the genes for two major antioxidant molecules— superoxide dismutase and catalase—were introduced into lines of the common fruit fly D. melanogaster. The amount of oxidative damage produced with age was reduced significantly in these lines, but, more important, both the average and maximum lifespans of the altered flies were increased by up to thirty percent.* Information was also gathered

---

*Interestingly, in a recent study, researchers in Toronto showed that the human gene for

in this study on metabolic potential. Metabolic potential refers to the total amount of oxygen consumed, and the energy produced from it, across an animal's entire lifespan. It is an indirect indicator of how much energy an animal has at its disposal to spend on pursuing its goals in life, whatever they may be. For some animals, lifespan may well be defined in terms of a total amount of energy generated and expended. We know, for example, that when lifespan is extended in cold-blooded animals simply by lowering the ambient temperature, the total amount of oxygen they consume in their extended lifetime at the lower temperature is about the same as that consumed in their briefer lifetime at the higher temperature. In these cold-blooded animals living at different temperatures, metabolic potential is a zero-sum game; they can live longer, but at a significantly reduced metabolic rate. Caloric restriction may be doing the same thing; reducing caloric intake almost certainly decreases the generation of oxidative waste products, but if it also decreases an individual's metabolic potential, the extended lifespan achieved may be partially offset by reduced metabolic capacity.

But in the Texas Drosophila study, the researchers found that in flies whose lifespan was increased by antioxidant supplementation, overall metabolic potential was actually increased. While metabolic rates in younger flies was about the same in treated and control groups, the older flies receiving antioxidants had a significantly higher metabolic potential than age-matched, untreated controls, suggesting that the extended lifespan observed was accompanied by an overall increase in metabolic activity. What these results suggest is that the lifespan benefit achieved with antioxidants does not necessarily have to come with a trade-off in terms of reduced metabolic activity; rather, the potential for activity in old age may actually be increased.

Almost certainly, oxidative damage to DNA is the major contributor to cellular senescence. The ability of animals to repair DNA damage as a function of age has been studied by a number of laboratories, often with conflicting results, but in general there is a tendency toward a decrease in the ability to repair radiation- or oxidation-induced DNA

---

superoxide dismutase can function in Drosophilia to give a similar increase in lifespan. This is one of the many examples of the tremendous evolutionary conservation of genes involved both in the generation of and in defenses against oxygen by-products.

damage, including telomere damage, with increasing age in many different cell types. In a recent study of DNA repair processes in human cells grown in vitro, the rate of accumulation of the type of chromosomal and DNA damage caused by oxidation (among other things) was assessed in normal human fibroblasts of different ages, and in cells taken from patients with Werner and Cockayne syndromes and other progeric disorders. There were clearly higher levels of abnormalities in the DNA and chromosomes from older patients and in the cells of progeric patients. DNA samples with purposely introduced oxidative damage were also injected into these cells; younger cells were able to repair the damage much more efficiently than older cells or progeric cells. The inability to repair DNA damage was found to correlate very well with the replicative capacity of these cells in vitro, suggesting a possible connection between oxidatively induced DNA damage and the phenomenon of replicative senescence.

Some of the most convincing evidence for a role of oxidative stress in determining lifespan comes from studies carried out in the nematode worm *C. elegans*. Certain mutations of the *C. elegans* gene age-1 can result in a near doubling of maximal lifespan. Worms with the age-1 mutation show increased resistance to both oxidative and thermal stress. Although the identity of the age-1 gene is not yet known, this mutation is accompanied by a decrease in the accumulation of DNA damage, an increase in the ability to repair ultraviolet-induced DNA alterations, and an increase in intracellular levels of antioxidant molecules such as superoxide dismutase and catalase.

The impact of caloric restriction on maximum lifespan as described in the last chapter is certainly interpretable in terms of the oxidative stress hypothesis. Oxygen radicals are produced as a direct result of "burning" foodstuffs to produce energy. If the amount of foodstuffs burned is kept to a minimum consistent with actual energetic needs, fewer oxygen radicals will be produced, which should be accompanied by reduced radical-mediated molecular damage. Animals kept on calorically restricted diets do in fact show significant reductions in the normal age-associated increases in generation of oxygen radicals by mitochondria and by systems such as cytochrome P450 in the liver. Calorically restricted animals also generally have enhanced levels of endogenous antioxidant enzymes. The greatest degree of oxidative damage is normally seen in hard-working tissues such as the brain and skeletal and cardiac muscle, and as we have seen damage to these tissues is greatly retarded in animals on calorically restricted diets.

The impact of caloric restriction on DNA repair in animals has also been studied by a number of researchers. The majority of these studies suggest that DNA repair is more efficient in animals maintained on a calorically restricted diet than in fully fed control animals. Most impressive is that the extensive damage to mitochondrial DNA with age is substantially retarded by caloric restriction. All of these observations are consistent with reduced oxidative damage as the explanation of caloric restriction. The flip side of the argument, that over-consumption of foodstuffs may actually reduce maximal lifespan, should then also be interpretable in terms of the over-production of oxidative damage.

Finally, the oxidative stress hypothesis of aging has direct implications for the theories of the evolution of senescence discussed in Chapter 3. Oxidative damage was present in eukaryotic cells as an internal danger from the moment they incorporated oxygen-metabolizing prokaryotes into their cellular life cycle. Oxidative damage now seems to be the major source of senescence-inducing damage in eukaryotic cells. Thus we do not need to look to rather complicated evolutionary theories to explain the acquisition of genes that cause senescence; a substantial number of them were incorporated into eukaryotic cells from the very beginning of their evolutionary history. The major task in the evolution of eukaryotes has been to develop means to deal with the damage wrought by oxygen radicals, forestalling senescence where necessary to allow different species to complete their reproductive cycle, yet allowing this damage to take its toll once reproduction has been achieved. While it seems likely that a few genes contributing to nonoxidative senescence have indeed crept into eukaryotic genomes over evolutionary time, it is likely that the contributions of these genes to senescence have been minor, and that the major senescence-inducing genes came in through the endosymbiosis of oxygen-using prokaryotes.

Oxidative Damage in Human Aging and Age-Related Disease

The data from in vivo animal studies and from the study of animal and human cells in vitro all strongly suggest a major role for oxidative damage in the aging of both organisms and cells. In fact everything we understand at present about senescence is consistent with the idea that oxidative damage is a likely primary cause of the aging process in animals. Are we ready, then, to conclude that oxidative stress is the key factor in aging and age-related diseases in human beings? The problem with drawing such a conclusion is that we cannot do the type of direct experiments on human beings required to establish this point with absolute certainty. We cannot, for example, deliberately expose human beings to excess oxidative damage and observe the effect this has on aging. The nature of the evidence we do have on this question is thus of necessity indirect. For example, data on the accumulation of oxidative products with aging and disease in the human body would support such a conclusion. There is a definite increase in serum levels of oxidative products in elderly individuals, and a decreased ability to generate natural antioxidants. In the cardiovascular disease that often accompanies normal aging, oxidative modification of the lipid-protein complex involved in removing cholesterol from the blood—low-density lipoprotein (LDL)—appears to be a major factor in the development of atherosclerotic plaques. Atherosclerotic plaques from elderly heart patients examined at autopsy also show a high level of oxidized lipids and high levels of the metal ions that promote oxidative reactions. These observations are all consistent with, but in fact do not demand, the conclusion that oxidative damage is a primary mechanism in human aging.

Although we cannot directly expose humans to greater or lesser amounts of oxidative damage, or to differing levels of antioxidant protection, individuals actually do this to themselves, largely through diet. Overeating, and in particular consumption of excess fat in the diet, places a major oxidative burden on virtually all the cells in our bodies. On the other hand, fruits and vegetables are excellent sources of natural antioxidants such as ascorbic acid (vitamin C), the tocopherols (vitamin E), and carotenoids (related to vitamin A). By and large, the effects of diet on aging and disease can be demonstrated only by the study of large populations. Such epidemiological studies have repeatedly shown that consumption of dietary antioxidants is associated with major reductions in age-related diseases. It is tempting to conclude, although perhaps not yet justified on the basis of presently available data, that consistent, long-term consumption of a diet rich in natural antioxidants retards the development of these diseases by retarding the natural aging process, and specifically cellular senescence.

There are a number of ongoing, large-scale epidemiological studies currently underway in the United States and many other countries in which large numbers of individuals voluntarily submit to exhaustive analyses of their life-style (including diet) and health. These individuals are then tracked over many years, with frequent updates of their profiles, to see which diseases they develop, how long they live, and what causes their death. One of the largest such studies in the United States is the Nurses Health Study, which has tracked over 120,000 women, with starting ages of thirty to fifty-five years, since 1976. The separate but closely related Health Professionals Study has tracked more than 50,000 males, with starting ages from forty to seventy-five years, since 1986. Another important study group is the Iowa Women's Health Study, which involves a random selection of just under 100,000 post-menopausal women aged fifty-five to sixty-nine years in 1985. Long-term studies of these magnitudes, with appropriate controls and statistical analysis of the data, are absolutely necessary to determine with any degree of confidence what effect diet or lifestyle has on any aspect of human health. All comparisons of dietary effects in studies with these population groups can be adjusted for other life-style attributes such as smoking. The fact that all information on dietary and other lifestyle habits is gathered before the onset of disease minimizes any possible bias relating to selection of individuals for the study of any particular disease or aging parameter.

In 1993, Dr. Bruce Ames published a paper in the prestigious Proceedings of the National Academy of Sciences summarizing the current state of knowledge about the effects of dietary and supplemental antioxidants on human disease and the aging process, as gathered from both basic science studies and large epidemiological studies of the type just described. He carefully marshaled the existing evidence supporting a role for oxidative damage in human maladies as wide-ranging as cardiovascular disease, cataracts, cancer, nervous disorders, and birth defects. In the same article, Dr. Ames also discussed the nature of the evidence that dietary antioxidants can have a significant effect on lowering the incidence and severity of many diseases and malfunctions associated with old age, including cancer, cardiovascular disease, cataracts, and neurological pathologies, among others. For example, he cited a monumental review of over 170 mostly smaller studies examining the relationship between diet and cancer. This study, published in the journal *Nutrition and Cancer*, showed a significant protective effect of fruit and vegetable consumption in 128 of 156 statistically interpretable cases. For most types of cancer, persons with the lowest fruit and vegetable intake had twice the cancer risk of persons with high intakes. Since that time, a large number of studies have confirmed Dr. Ames's contention that many of the major age-related diseases in humans are strongly associated with, and very likely caused by, oxidative cellular damage.

Vitamin E and Breast Cancer

Vitamin E is a complex of eight different lipophilic (fat-loving) compounds, some of which, particularly alpha-tocopherol, have been shown in animal studies to be highly effective antioxidants. These compounds usually insert into a cell's membranes, from where they actively scavenge reactive oxidative molecules. Vitamin E is found in mitochondrial membranes, for example, and presumably aids in mopping up escaped oxygen radicals at the site of generation. The efficacy of vitamin E is dependent on an adequate dietary source of selenium. Vitamin E also interacts with vitamin C; the latter acts somewhat like a recharger, removing some of the reactive oxygen molecules from vitamin E to itself, thereby releasing "recharged" vitamin E to scavenge again. Like all vitamins, vitamin E cannot be made by the body and must be obtained from food or taken as a vitamin supplement. Unfortunately, vitamin E is found only in fatty foods such as oils, nuts, and shortenings, which are avoided by many people for general health reasons, and which are thought to be especially problematic for women at risk for breast cancer. It has long been recognized, for example, that Japanese women living in Japan, where dietary fat is unusually low, have a very low breast cancer rate. However, when these women migrate to the United States or other Western countries with high-fat diets, their breast cancer rates rapidly approach that of women in the host country. This puts women between the proverbial rock and a hard place: Avoiding a known risk factor for breast cancer—fatty foods—deprives them of a natural source of a potent cancer-fighting antioxidant—vitamin E.

At least two dozen studies have now shown that vitamin E given in supplemental form to rats and mice that develop spontaneous breast tumors significantly reduces the onset and severity of their cancers. Vitamin E has also been shown to interfere with the growth of human breast cancer cells grown in vitro, and to ameliorate breast tenderness in women prone to benign cysts. Epidemiological studies, summarized in a recent issue of the journal *Nutrition and Cancer*, also support a role for vitamin E in reducing breast cancer, although the data at this stage is not particularly strong. Because of the great variation in the design of the ten studies analyzed, some of which depended on patient recall of dietary habits over a number of years, and varying intakes of dietary versus supplemental vitamin E, the precise relationship between vitamin E and breast cancer is difficult to discern. Nevertheless, a positive effect was seen in eight of ten studies, and in several of these the protective effect was quite strong. More precisely controlled studies will likely be planned for the future. In the meantime, because the animal and in vitro studies are so strong, and since vitamin E is essentially nontoxic in humans, even at high doses, it has been suggested that women in general should make every effort to assure they receive generous amounts of this vitamin through their diets, and that women especially at risk for breast cancer may want to consider taking supplemental vitamin E as well.

Antioxidant Vitamins and Cardiovascular Disease

As with the effects of antioxidants on cancer, there is a strong basis in animal studies and epidemiological analyses to support the notion that antioxidants can lower the risk of atherosclerosis and cardiovascular disease in humans. Vitamin E has been shown in studies with chickens, rabbits, and monkeys, as well as rats and mice, to have a marked inhibitory effect on the development of atherosclerotic lesions. Vitamin E actually associates with the LDL complex, inhibiting the oxidation that is associated with atherosclerotic plaques. In some animal studies, vitamin C and carotenoids such as beta carotene have also been shown to provide protection against atherosclerosis.

There is also suggestive evidence from studies of dietary habits in humans indicating a positive effect of antioxidant vitamins on heart disease; again, those consuming high levels of fresh fruits and vegetables had a lower incidence of cardiovascular disease. Two European studies also showed that high serum concentrations of vitamin E were correlated with a lower incidence of heart disease, and vice versa. The evidence for protective effects of vitamin C and carotenoids was less clear. In addition to vitamins, antioxidant drugs also have a strong protective effect against cardiovascular disease. One of the earliest cholesterol-lowering drugs, Probucol, is a strong antioxidant that, like vitamin E, physically associates with LDL, inhibiting the atherosclerosis-promoting oxidative damage that results in improper uptake of cholesterol into cells.

Studies using very large numbers of human subjects, such as those provided by the Nurses Health Study, the Iowa Women's Study, and the Health Professionals Study, generally support the earlier studies. In the Nurses Health Study it was found that those individuals with the highest vitamin E intake had a 34 percent reduction in cardiovascular disease. Most of the women in this highest-intake group were also taking supplementary vitamin E. High beta carotene intake was associated with a 22 percent reduction in cardiovascular disease, but because of the small numbers (552 total cases of heart disease in the population base), this effect is only marginally statistically significant.The effect of vitamin C was also statistically uncertain. In the Health Professionals Study, both vitamin E and beta carotene showed modest protective effects; vitamin C showed no effect at all. In the Iowa Womens Study, which looked at cardiovascular mortality (as opposed to simple presence of disease), vitamin E was associated with a very strong decrease in mortality; carotenoids and vitamin C showed no correlation with deaths from cardiovascular disease. Several trials in which large numbers of individuals have been randomly assigned to supplements of antioxidant vitamins are now under way, and will eventually produce the most definitive results of all. However, at present it is too early in these trials to gain any clear impressions of what the results may tell us.

The evidence, both direct and indirect, that oxidative damage is a major factor in the development of age-related diseases, including not only cancer and heart disease but also kidney disease, cataracts, and more benign problems such as degeneration of skin and muscle, is quite compelling. At present we cannot say with complete certainty that individuals consuming diets high in antioxidants, or taking supplemental antioxidants, will live longer. The answer to that question will likely emerge from the large-scale epidemiological studies and direct supplementation trials currently under way, but will certainly take many years. Reducing mortality from heart disease and cancer would be expected to have at least a modest effect on average lifespan.

There are other questions about oxidative damage and lifespan that remain unanswered. For example, oxygen consumption increases enormously during vigorous exercise, and would be expected to generate additional reactive oxygen species. Does there come a point in life when a decreased ability to neutralize oxygen radicals might outweigh the proven advantages of strenuous exercise? Can this be offset by antioxidant supplementation? We simply do not know at present whether excess oxygen consumption in the elderly is dangerous or whether it could be controlled by antioxidants. We would also like to know a great deal more about why antioxidants taken in with food appear to be so much more effective than highly purified vitamins taken supplementally. Are there as-yet unidentified elements in foodstuffs that increase the effectiveness of the vitamins themselves? Could these "co-factors" be taken supplementally as well? We do not yet know, but one can be certain this question is being looked at very closely by nutritional supply companies.

Nevertheless, the evidence for the overall benefits of dietary and supplemental antioxidants, albeit largely indirect, is sufficiently strong at present that many health care professionals and nutritional experts are themselves reassessing their own diets, and where appropriate— when the individual is at risk for heart disease or breast cancer, for example—taking supplemental antioxidants, particularly vitamin E. The end of this story is not entirely clear, but its general outlines should begin to emerge in the next dozen years or so. It is a story with tremendous potential for human health, and one we should all watch very closely indeed.

10

The Aging Brain

One of the greatest fears associated with aging is the possibility that senescence may rob us of our mental faculties, leaving us to wander the empty spaces of our minds with none of the familiar landmarks that tell us where we are or where we have been. Each human personality is shaped by a unique combination of intellectual and emotional capacities, developed over a lifetime of learning and feeling, and exercised with a particular brand of reason and judgment that leads to a highly individualized response to the surrounding world. We each have our own way of seeing that world, of thinking about it and responding to it—of being in it—drawing upon a totally idiosyncratic collection of memories and experience. It is this personal collection that we label "self" and use to guide ourselves through our daily lives.

We connect our sense of who we are with our minds, but the mind is ultimately a product of the brain, largely of the outer regions of the brain known as the cerebral cortex. It is there, throughout most of our lifetime, that we spin the complex tapestry that makes each of us who we are. The threads of this tapestry are the nerve cells, or neurons, tied together in patterns of seemingly impenetrable complexity. Beginning even before we are born, and for a short while after birth, the neurons begin generating enormous numbers of nerve fibers that they simply cast out in the general direction of tissues and cells needing nerve connections. If a particular nerve fiber happens to find a cell with a nerve attachment point on its surface—another nerve cell, for example, or a muscle cell—it makes a connection. That fiber, and the neuron from which it came, will survive and become the nervous system's physical link with the targeted cell for life. If, on the other hand, the nerve fiber fails to establish contact with an appropriate cell—and fewer than half do—the neuron that sent it out must commit suicide, dying the same quiet apoptotic death that helped shape the developing hand (Fig. 2.1).

But gradually, as we age, this process reverses itself. Starting somewhere after the reproductive years have ended, with differing speeds and to differing extents in different individuals, senescence begins to take its toll in the brain and in the nervous system, just as it does in every other cell in the body, and many of the neural connections established over a lifetime of pattern weaving are broken. The cells will pull in their fibers and disconnect from one another. This process happens much more slowly in people who remain mentally and physically active—one of the more poignant manifestations of the adage "use it or lose it." Neuronal loss is itself only rarely a cause of organismal death in the normal aging process, but depending on how far the process advances before death comes, it can greatly diminish the quality of our remaining years.

Disruption of intercellular connections among the ten billion or so neurons forming the human brain is, however, a major cause of the gradual diminution of mental function that normally accompanies aging. Some degree of neural degeneration is detectable at autopsy in almost every person over sixty years of age. The type of degeneration neurons undergo is shown in Figure 10.1. Nerve impulses are brought into the cell by the relatively short fibers known as dendrites. Each neuron can have dozens of dendrites feeding information into it, and each dendrite is extensively branched at its tip, ultimately gathering information from a dozen or more different nerve cells. Each neuron may thus receive input from hundreds of other nerve cells. The neuron in turn sends information to other cells through its single outgoing fiber, the axon, which can be quite long and may also be branched at the tip, allowing connection with numerous other cells. If a nerve cell make its connection with another neuron, it normally does so by linking one of its axonal processes with that cell's dendrite, although occasionally a nerve cell may attach its axon directly to the cell body of another neuron. Nerve cells send and receive impulses by the release and uptake of special neural transmitters, small chemical molecules such as acetylcholine, stored in the tip of each axon. When appropriately stimulated, axons release these chemicals, which are picked up by the cell to which the axon is connected across a special structure called a synapse.

As neurons age they undergo a number of distinct intracellular changes (Fig. 10.1). One very characteristic alteration is the accumulation of lipofuscin, a dense, granular material composed mostly of oxidized lipids. The origin of this material is uncertain; it is presumed to be a storage form of lipids damaged by the oxidative wastes of metabolism. It has been a component of aging cells throughout much of eukaryotic evolution; even cells of the tiny nematode worm *C. elegans* accumulate lipofuscin with age, as do the post-mitotic cells making up insects such as fruit flies. As far as can be determined, lipofuscin gran-

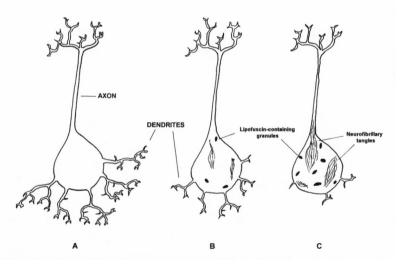

Figure 10.1. Intracellular changes in neurons during aging. As normal neurons (*A*) begin to age, they accumulate increasing amounts of lipofuscin, and begin to develop neurofibrillary tangles. The dendrites begin to degenerate (*B, C*), disrupting connections with other neurons. The neuron shown in *C* is probably very near death.

ules cause no harm to nerve cells. The same is not true of the neurofibrillary tangles, another characteristic inclusion of aging neurons.
These are twisted strands of protein that condense together inside the
cell, forming insoluble complexes often described as "flame-like." The
presence of neurofibrillary tangles in nerve cells is thought to be a sign
that the cell will soon die.

As a neuron begins to die, the most obvious change is a degeneration and pulling back of its dendrites. Very slowly, over a number of
years late in life, the number of dendrites feeding into nerve cells, and
the number of branches on the remaining dendrites, diminishes, and
the cells begin the slow slide toward death. Cell death contributes to
an actual decrease in brain weight, which can be 10 percent or more in
very old individuals. Overall brain volume does not change apprecia-
bly; the brain still sits snugly in its skull case. As the neurons disappear,
the fluid-filled spaces within the brain simply expand to fill the space.
The loss of neurons is not uniform throughout the brain. Some areas,
such as the cerebral cortex in a healthy, active older person, are only
marginally affected; other areas, such as the substantia nigra or the
locus ceruleus, may lose a third or more of their neurons in most individuals over eighty. These losses are often associated with problems
such as an inability to sleep or disorders such as Parkinson's disease, as
well as a gradual impairment of the ability to learn and remember. Premature or excessive neuronal loss is one of the hallmarks of Alzheimer's
disease, as we shall see. In the spinal cord, there is also a loss of neurons, particularly the motor neurons, which may interfere with movement and balance.

The brain is a classic example of an organ in the body where replicative senescence is unlikely to play a role in aging and age-associated
disease. Once neurons begin making connections with other neurons,
or with cells elsewhere in the body, they never divide again. The brain
is a post-mitotic organ, and it is obvious why this must be so. A fully
engaged neuron may have dozens, or even hundreds, of interconnections with other cells. For a brain cell to divide, it would have to break
each of these connections, undergo mitosis, and then try to find and
reform each of these connections. Aside from the "down-time" of that
neuron's function, which could likely be ill-afforded, the possibility of
finding all of the right connections after cell division would be
extremely small. From this it is also evident why damaged nerve tissue

can never be regenerated; there is no way a new nerve cell could find and make each of the connections established by the cell it would be replacing.

Alzheimer's Disease

The degeneration seen in the brain and nervous system with age are normally accompanied by definite but relatively minor cognitive deficits, such as loss of short-term memory, decreased stimulus-response times, and occasional mild confusion. When these problems begin to interfere seriously with an aging individual's social or work environment, we enter into the gray area of senile dementia. Dementia is defined as the loss of some combination of intellect and emotion, memory and judgment, without a loss of consciousness and the simpler cognitive functions, but with a detectable impairment of occupational or social function. "Senile" simply defines this loss as age-related. Perhaps two-thirds of senile dementias are attributable to some degree of Alzheimer's disease. Some Parkinson's disease patients also experience a form of dementia quite similar to Alzheimer's. Another common cause of dementia in the elderly is multiple infarct dementia, which results from the gradual destruction of tiny portions of the brain caused by recurrent, often undetected, small strokes. States of dementia not related to senility can usually be traced to particular drugs or drug combinations, microbial infections such as HIV, or other psychological states such as depression and stress; these reversible dementias often go away when the underlying cause is treated or removed.

The first report of what would become known as Alzheimer's disease was published by the German neuropathologist Alois Alzheimer in 1907, who described the findings at autopsy of a woman who had died at age fifty-five. Prior to death, she had suffered a progressive dementia involving severe memory, behavior, and language deficits. Alzheimer took advantage of recently developed histological stains based on the use of silver to examine the brain tissue of this patient, and he reported what was at the time a new finding: the presence, within the nerve cells themselves, of silver-staining structures that came to be known as the neurofibrillary tangles (Fig. 10.1 C). This patient also had an abnormally large loss of brain tissue, and the presence of numerous neuritic plaques composed of dead and dying nerve cells. Because of the relatively young age of the patient, Alzheimer's disease became the standard definition of presenile dementia (dementia setting in before sixty years of age) in the years immediately following his report. Alzheimer's initial three findings—neurofibrillary tangles, neuritic plaques, and marked tissue loss, leading to eventual death—are still the signature findings in all Alzheimer's patients.

There are today five million people in the United States diagnosed with Alzheimer's disease; current estimates are that about half of all persons over eighty-five have some degree of disease. It acounts for nearly 100,000 deaths annually in the United States. Based on the timing of onset of the disease, and to some extent on the underlying defect, Alzheimer's falls into two distinct categories. Approximately 95 percent of cases are late-onset Alzheimer's disease. This form of the disease arises from defects occurring in the individual within his or her life history, beginning any time after conception, and is not passed on to the individual's offspring. About 5 percent of Alzheimer's cases are of the inherited type, and are characterized by early onset of disease symptoms—before sixty years of age. Yet even this early form of Alzheimer's occurs after the reproductive period of an individual's life, allowing the genes to be passed on to the next generation. Late-onset Alzheimer's disease is becoming of increasing sociological concern, because it affects a significant portion of what is the fastest growing segment of the population in industrialized countries; those eighty-five years of age or older. Current demographic trends indicate that the number of people severely disabled by Alzheimer's disease will double every twenty years during the next century. Barring discovery of an effective treatment or cure, the impact on health care costs will be enormous. The burden on families who must care for these seriously and distressingly incapacitated individuals will be equally catastrophic.

Defining the relation of Alzheimer's disease to normal aging of the brain has posed a major challenge to neurologists since it was first described. Human average lifespan has increased substantially since Alzheimer's first patient, and so the presence of Alzheimer's-type lesions in very old individuals, without the disabling dementia typical of fully developed Alzheimer's disease, took some time to be appreciated. The picture was clarified somewhat in the 1950s when other causes of dementia, such as multiple cerebral infarcts, drugs, and depression, were clearly identified. Still, even when only the more "classical" Alzheimer's cases are considered, their relationship to normal aging is not always clear. Loss of brain tissue and the presence of neurofibrillary tangles are seen to some extent in most people over sixty. Even neuritic plaques are seen in people who live long enough— beyond age eighty or so. They are simply seen earlier, in the case of presenile dementia, or develop to an exaggerated degree that can lead to death, in elderly people with clinically verified late-onset Alzheimer's disease. Histologically, there is no difference in the tangles and plaques seen in normally aging brain and those found in Alzheimer's disease patients. It is possible, however, that the patterns of distribution of damaged cells within the brain is slightly different in normal aging and in Alzheimer's disease.

Thus the difference between the neurological changes seen in normal aging and those seen in Alzheimer's disease may be as much quantitative as qualitative. Unfortunately, there is no simple test at present that can definitively establish the presence of Alzheimer's disease, so the diagnosis depends on the physician's assessment of the degree of loss of cognitive function, and on ruling out other possible causes of that loss. The changes in cognitive function characterizing Alzheimer's disease include severe memory loss and impairment of language skills, learning ability, and the ability to think abstractly and make reasonable judgments about events in one's surroundings. Other symptoms include fearfulness, delusions, excessive irritability, and unusual aggressive behavior. While all of these traits may appear to some degree with age in everyone, it is only when they seriously interfere with an individual's ability to function in his or her daily life that a tentative diagnosis of Alzheimer's disease is made. When followed by critical laboratory tests and a detailed neurological examination, the accuracy of diagnosis is now about 90 percent, but a truly definitive diagnosis can only be made at postmortem examination.

It was apparent early on that the number of neurofibrillary tangles found at autopsy correlates well with the severity of the disease during the patient's lifetime, and it is now generally agreed that neurofibrillary tangles are intimately involved in the pathology of Alzheimer's disease. The quantity of neurofibrillary tangles within cells is much greater in individuals diagnosed with Alzheimer's disease than in age- and sex-matched individuals without this disease. The neurofibrillary tangles found in normally aged brains are thus presumed to be involved in the normal mental deficits of old age. They are composed mostly of the so-called tau protein, which is found in association with the cytoskeleton, the proteinaceous framework that gives a cell its shape and assists it in moving around. Why these proteins show up in neurofibrillary tangles is something of a mystery. The tau proteins wind around one another in very tight helices, which take up silver stains and are the flame-shaped structures within affected cells (Fig. 10.1). This process may be promoted by excess aluminum within the cells, although this is still a controversial point. The exact cellular events that trigger formation of neurofibrillary tangles are simply not understood at present.

The presence of neuritic plaques, sometimes called senile plaques, is a sign of severe neuronal degeneration and loss. Neuritic plaques are occasionally seen in normal aged brains, but only in the oldest old individuals. They are very common in Alzheimer's disease. The plaques are found in highest concentration in the so-called "associational areas" of the brain. Neurons in these areas have extensive interconnections with neurons in other parts of the brain—connections presumably involved in the coordination of mental functions related to intellect, judgment, and memory. These neurons are particularly important in the sorting and storage of short-term memories, such as recently learned names or telephone numbers. Some of these neurons, called pyramidal neurons, are much larger than normal brain cells and have a great many more intercellular connections with other neurons; these are the cells most subject to degeneration. The regions of the brain involved with sensory perception and motor functions are only marginally affected. The few viable neurons that may be found within neuritic plaques are largely devoid of dendrites, and may also show axonal deformity.

As with neurofibrillary tangles, the severity of Alzheimer's disease correlates strongly with the number of neuritic plaques found in the brain at autopsy. Whereas the tangles probably identify nerve cells that will soon die, the plaques are essentially open gravesites filled with dead neurons. It is assumed that continued fusion of neuritic plaques is a major cause factor in creation of the empty regions of the brain characteristic of advanced Alzheimer's disease.

Each neuritic plaque contains not only large numbers of dead and dying cells, but also deposits of amyloid protein. Deposition of amyloid protein is not limited to Alzheimer's disease and to the brain. It commonly occurs as one concomitant of the replicative senescence of fibroblasts grown in vitro. Accumulation of amyloid deposits in vivo, or amyloidosis, is a condition that arises under a variety of circumstances. Amyloidosis associated with aging involves many tissues in addition to the brain, in particular the heart and the pancreas. Amyloid deposition also occurs in connection with particular diseases and is often found in chronic inflammatory states. There is no single amyloid protein characterizing all of these lesions, but the proteins involved in all of them are polymerized into insoluble fibers and share common reactions with certain chemical stains used to detect them. The significance of amyloid deposits is likely different in each of the situations where they are found. The particular form of amyloid protein found in the brain is referred to as beta-amyloid protein. In addition to neuritic plaques, beta amyloid protein is also found deposited in blood vessels serving the brain, which is thought to contribute to the overall pathology associated with normal aging, perhaps in the form of so-called "microstrokes" that damage tiny portions of the brain, as well as with full-blown Alzheimer's disease.

Genetics of Alzheimer's Disease

Inheritance patterns of Alzheimer's disease have long been of interest to geneticists. The majority of cases are of the late-onset type, and are traditionally referred to as either familial or sporadic Alzheimer's disease. In so-called sporadic Alzheimer's, there is no obvious pattern of familial inheritance, and the disease is presumed to have arisen spontaneously within the individual. In familial Alzheimer's disease, there is a tendency for a higher frequency of disease within certain family lineages, but the nature of the genes involved is not always clear. A genetic element in late-onset Alzheimer's is suggested by the fact that there is anywhere from 50 to 80 percent (depending on the study) concordance of late-onset disease in genetically identical twins, whereas concordance in fraternal twins of the same sex ranges from 20 to 40 percent. On the other hand, the fact that the concordance is not 100 percent in identical twins, plus the fact that the age of onset even in identical twins can vary by a dozen years, suggests environmental factors must also play an important role.

Although the distinction between "familial" and "sporadic"

Alzheimer's disease is a long-standing one, it is not entirely clear that the distinction is real. The apparent clustering of Alzheimer's disease in certain families could well be due to the fact that people in these families live longer; given that Alzheimer's is fairly common in the oldest old, families in which members frequently reach a very old age might appear to have a rather higher frequency of the disease. On the other hand, in families where members die at earlier ages from other causes, there may appear to be little or no Alzheimer's disease. It might not be Alzheimer's disease per se that is inherited in these families, but rather a tendency for longer average lifespan.

On the other hand, a small number of cases of Alzheimer's disease—perhaps no more than 3 to 5 percent—are clearly caused by mutations in one of several possible autosomal-dominant genes. These cases are almost always of the early-onset type (forty-five to sixty years of age), probably similar to the case seen by Alzheimer himself at the beginning of this century. Inheritance patterns and specific gene associations for early-onset disease are quite strong. The pathology of this type of disease is not significantly different from the late-onset form; the difference appears to be restricted to the timing of onset. So far three genes have been implicated that, when mutated in specific ways, can result in early-onset Alzheimer's disease. One of these genes had been traced some years ago to chromosome 21, which was of great interest because that is the chromosome involved in Down's syndrome. This syndrome is sometimes referred to as "trisomy-21 disorder," because those afflicted with it have three rather than the normal two copies of chromosome 21. Down's syndrome patients who survive to age thirty-five or so always show evidence of Alzheimer's disease, both clinically and at postmortem examination.

The chromosome 21 gene is called APP, because it encodes a protein called amyloid precursor protein. The APP protein is found embedded in the membranes of all cells in the body. Its normal cellular function is not known, but its synthesis and processing in cells, critical to understanding the pathology of Alzheimer's disease, are known in some detail (Fig. 10.2). APP is a protein composed of 726 amino acids. After insertion into the cell membrane, APP is cleaved at amino acid 671, liberating a soluble, smaller protein of 45 amino acids called APP_s. (The rest of the molecule remains inserted in the cell membrane.) APP_s is an intermediate molecule that is normally further

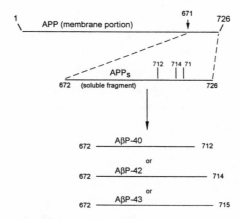

Figure 10.2. Processing of the APP protein to produce AßP molecules of various lengths.

modified to produce a 40-amino-acid final soluble product called AßP.

Alzheimer's disease can be caused by overproduction of APP itself or by mutations in the APP gene that result in the production of slightly longer versions of AßP. Overproduction of normal APP appears to cause Alzheimer's symptoms and pathology in Down's syndrome, and overexpression of the APP gene in brain cells cultured in vitro has been shown to result in the buildup of AßP-containing deposits, resulting in neuronal cell death. Mice given an extra APP gene develop severe Alzheimer's-like brain pathology. In early-onset disease, specific mutations in the APP gene result in a change in the processing of APP_s that results in the production of AßP molecules containing either 41 or 42 amino acids, rather than the normal 40. These slightly longer molecules condense more readily into multistranded amyloid sheets that form the bulk of the material found in neuritic plaques. Although the 40-amino-acid version of AßP can also form amyloid sheets and cause disease when it is overproduced, the 41- and 42-amino-acid forms cause earlier and more aggressive disease. It may seem extraordinary that such a minor change in the processing of a protein could have such disastrous consequences, but the body's chemistry is extremely fine-tuned.

Mutations in the APP gene turn out to account for only a minor portion of early-onset disease. By far the majority of cases involve mutations in two additional genes, discovered only in the past few years, called presenilin-1 (PS-1; mapping to chromosome 14) and presenilin-2 (PS-2; found on chromosome 1). These two genes are closely related, sharing 67 percent amino-acid sequence homology in the corresponding proteins. Over thirty mutations have been found in PS-1; only two have been found so far in PS-2. The PS-1 mutations account for roughly three-quarters of early-onset cases. Disease induced by PS-2 is more rare, and appears to be milder and slightly later in setting in.

As with APP, mutations in the presenilins are dominant and fully penetrant, meaning that only one of the two gene copies need be mutated, and the presence of an appropriate mutation results in a 100 percent certainty of disease. The presence of such mutations results in exactly the same phenotype as APP mutations—production of slightly longer forms of AßP and development of Alzheimer's disease. The proteins encoded by these two genes are, like the APP protein, membrane-bound and found in all cells in the body. As with APP, the normal function of these proteins is unknown. It is also not known how mutations in these genes cause the production of longer AßP molecules or why the addition of one or two amino acids to AßP should enhance its precipitation in neuritic plaques. Although mutations in any of the three genes discussed above can trigger early-onset Alzheimer's disease, 10 percent or so of presenile Alzheimer's patients do not show mutations in any of the three, so presumably there are additional genes waiting to be discovered.

Although we do not yet understand exactly what PS-1 and -2 do in the body under normal circumstances, some intriguing clues have come from studies carried out in the roundworm *C. elegans*. One of the great advantages of *C. elegans* for understanding the function of the human body is that nematodes and humans are about as far apart evolutionarily as any two multicellular organisms could be, having diverged at least 800 million years ago. Therefore, whenever we find genes that are highly conserved between these two species, it suggests the genes are encoding extremely important functions, functions too important to have been tampered with during evolution.

It turns out that *C. elegans* has a gene called sel-12 that has approximately 50 percent homology with human PS-1 and -2. The sel-12 gene is involved in the embryonic development of several tissues in *C. elegans*, including nervous system tissue. The equivalent genes have also been identified in mice, and were found to be expressed very strongly in the mouse brain during embryonic development, but at very low levels in the adult brain. Recently, "knockout mice" lacking the PS-1 gene were created and mated to see whether they could produce viable offspring. The embryos of these mice barely survived until birth; although the cellular architecture of the brain appeared normal, there was extensive hemorrhaging in both the brain and spinal cord, suggesting that PS-1 and -2 may be important in developing nervous system vasculature. Given the close parallels in human and mouse embryonic development, it seems likely that these genes play a similar role in development of the human brain.

How defects in brain vasculature might translate into the defects seen in Alzheimer's disease later in life is unclear, but further studies of these genes and their proteins in lower animals will likely shed light on this question. And it is quite possible that the answer may be unveiled in *C. elegans* itself. The fact that the majority of PS-1 mutations resulting in early-onset Alzheimer's disease affect amino acids evolutionarily conserved in PS-1 and sel-12 led researchers to ask whether the two genes might play functionally identical roles in these two widely separated species. This turns out to be the case. One of the phenotypes produced in *C. elegans* as a result of sel-12 mutations affects the ability to lay eggs. Researchers have used human PS-1 genes in a form of "gene therapy" to try to correct the *C. elegans* defect. When normal forms of human PS-1 were introduced, the defect in *C. elegans* was completely repaired. However, when forms of PS-1 that lead to Alzheimer's disease were tested, the ability to correct the sel-12 defect was greatly reduced or absent. This suggests that PS-1 and sel-12 almost certainly are involved in the same fundamental cellular role in humans and in *C. elegans*, and that a detailed analysis of sel-12 function in nematodes will very likely provide important insights into the function of PS-1 in humans.

In the inherited form of Alzheimer's disease, by definition the same mutations must be present in every cell of the body, and presumably the longer forms of AßP caused by mutations in any of these three genes are produced throughout the body. Yet the condensation of these longer forms into plaques containing dead cells occurs only in the brain. There is some laboratory evidence suggesting that the longer AßP molecules are directly and selectively toxic to nerve cells, which would be an attractive explanation of neuritic plaques, but this remains to be confirmed.

The existence of allelic variants of the APP, PS-1, and PS-2 genes that cause early-onset Alzheimer's disease are obvious candidates for senescence effector genes. Clearly they are genetically fixed in the human species, and so at some point must have been seen by evolution and natural selection as somehow advantageous. Perhaps this advantage still exists today, although no one has any idea what it might be, since we really do not know the function of the underlying gene itself. Given that the negative effects of these alleles are seen only in post-reproductive individuals, who would have been an exceedingly small part of the species until very recently, no negative pressure against the selection of these alleles would have been exercised. As other causes of death were gradually brought under control, the contribution of the heritable forms of Alzheimer's disease have become significant contributors to "natural death" caused by senescence.

The genetic basis for the late-onset forms of Alzheimer's disease is less clear. So far there is little evidence for an involvement of the three genes responsible for early-onset disease. But since there is no evidence that Alzheimer's disease is triggered by outside agents, it is reasonable to suspect the involvement of faulty endogenous genes. Since 1991, it has been suspected from a study of family lineages that a heritable gene located on chromosome 19 may be involved in late-onset disease. One gene located on chromosome 19, called ApoE, was identified in 1993, and is altered in over 70 percent of cases of late-onset disease. This gene was identified in a completely different manner than the gene identified through family studies, and it is unclear whether the two genes are the same. ApoE encodes a protein that is involved in the transport of fat (lipid) molecules through the bloodstream. Fat molecules are not soluble in water-based blood, and on their own would have a tendency to stick to the walls of blood vessels. Certain proteins, while water-soluble themselves, have "lipid-friendly" regions that can bind to lipid molecules and carry them to move through the bloodstream without causing problems. The ApoE protein, for example, is part of the complex called LDL, which helps transport cholesterol through the blood. Interestingly, the heritable variant of ApoE that confers high risk for Alzheimer's disease—epsilon 4 (ε4)—is the same variant that is a recognized risk factor in heart disease and stroke.

It turns out that the ApoE protein is also able to bind to AßP molecules; whether this is through the same binding site ApoE uses to bind lipids is not clear at present. Intriguingly, however, ApoE binds to the same site on AßP that AßP molecules use to bind to each other in forming the insoluble amyloid sheets associated with neuritic plaques. There are three different alleles of the ApoE gene in the population, called ε2, ε3, and ε4 (see Table 10.1). Some 60 percent of the population in the United States has two copies of the ε3 allele (i.e., is ε3/ε3). The ε4 allele binds most tightly to AßP, and among late-onset Alzheimer's patients the frequency of this allele is twice as high as in age-matched control groups. Statisticians have calculated that someone with two ε4 alleles (i.e., someone who is ε4/ε4; 2 to 3 percent of the U.S. population) is three times as likely to develop late-onset Alzheimer's disease as someone with no ε4 alleles.

Interestingly, the frequency of ε4 in healthy centenarians is half that in younger people; presumably, those individuals with ε4 succumbed to Alzheimer's or other ε4-mediated diseases at an earlier age. On the other hand, the ε2 allele is generally viewed as protective, in that persons with ε2 alleles are less likely even than those with ε3 to develop Alzheimer's disease. In those rare cases when disease does set in in persons carrying ε2, it is usually later and more mild than in persons lacking ε2. As might be expected, ε2 is much more frequent in centenarians than in younger individuals. Almost exactly the same pattern is seen in atherosclerosis—ε4 being a risk factor and ε2 being protective—suggesting the underlying biology may be similar.

Some studies show that individuals with two ε4 alleles develop their disease earlier and have more neurofibrillary tangles and neuritic plaques. As with the genes involved in early-onset disease, we do not know exactly how the ε4 allele causes disease symptoms. Clearly, the ε4 allele of the ApoE gene cannot be thought of as causative for Alzheimer's disease in the same way that certain alleles of the APP,

Table 10.1. *ApoE allele frequencies in patient and control populations*

	E2	E3	E4
Control population	.08	.77	.22
Early-onset Alzheimer's disease	.06	.61	.33
Late-onset Alzheimer's disease	.03	.51	.46

PS-1, and PS-2 genes are causative for early onset disease. Inheritance of any of the latter variants is accompanied by complete certainty of developing the disease; inheritance of ε4 is recognized as a risk factor, but apparently ε4 must interact with other, as yet identified factors—genetic or environmental—to cause disease. Moreover, some ε4/ε4 individuals do not develop Alzheimer's symptoms at all, and about a third of late-onset disease occurs in individuals lacking even one ε4 allele. Given that the pathology of early- and late-onset disease is essentially identical, and that all early-onset disease is related to inappropriate processing of APP, many are looking to this pathway for an explanation of late-onset disease as well. On the other hand, it is entirely possible that ApoE does not play a direct causative role in Alzheimer's disease per se. It has been suggested that its normal function may be in repairing normally occurring damage to neurons; ε4 would then be seen as a particularly inefficient variant of a needed repair protein.

Oxidative Stress and Aging in the Brain

As with cellular aging in so many other regions of the body, there is increasing evidence that oxidative stress plays a major role in the senescence of brain cells, in both normal aging and Alzheimer's disease. As in other cells, the major targets of oxidative damage in the brain are proteins, DNA, and the lipids found in cellular membranes. Researchers have noted for a dozen years or more an age-related increase in oxidatively damaged molecules, particularly lipids, in the human brain. Oxidative damage to DNA (especially mitochondrial DNA) is up to three-fold higher in brain samples from Alzheimer's patients and is substantially increased in very old patients without clinically detectable disease. There is also an age-dependent increase in endogenous antioxidant enzymes, in an apparent attempt by neurons to deal with the oxidative challenge.

One theory of how oxidative damage is generated in neuritic plaques focuses on the oxidative properties of AßP. Studies with highly purified synthetic AßP have shown that it is capable of reacting with oxygen dissolved in water (the form of oxygen present in extracellular fluids, where AßP is found), and that dissolved oxygen is necessary to generate the ß-amyloid sheets that are a characteristic feature of neuritic plaques. The oxygen radicals generated by the interaction of AßP with molecular oxygen could then damage surrounding neurons, hastening their death. In fact, damage very similar to that caused by AßP in cultures of nerve cells can be reproduced by adding oxidants such as hydrogen peroxide to the cultures, and the damage by AßP is at least partially reversible by antioxidants. Another source of oxidative damage is thought to be phagocytes attracted to the neuritic plaques by the large numbers of dead and dying cells; oxygen radicals spilled during the "cleaning-up" process engaged in by phagocytes surrounding and infiltrating neuritic plaques could further exacerbate the damage. The damage caused by AßP-generated oxygen radicals would be additive with any oxidative damage generated within nerve cells themselves as a concomitant of aging. Thus damage triggered by AßP would essentially accelerate a normal endogenous process, consistent with our view of what Alzheimer's disease represents. All forms of Alzheimer's disease described so far involve in one way or another a perturbation in the processing of APP to AßP.

That oxidative damage might contribute to neuronal degradation has been supported by numerous studies in experimental animals. A detailed study in gerbils showed that as these animals age, there is an increase in the levels of oxidized proteins in their brain tissues. This age-related increase could be prevented, and even reversed, by treatment of the animals over time with a potent antioxidant called PBN. That this reversal had functional significance was demonstrated in a so-called radial maze test, which analyzes spatial and temporal learning and memory. Young gerbils made an average of four mistakes in working their way through this maze problem. Old gerbils made eight mistakes on average in the same test. But old gerbils that had been maintained on PBN not only had less oxidative brain damage, but they made only four mistakes in the maze test. That the effect of the PBN was truly on an age-dependent change in the older animals was shown by the fact that the number of mistakes made by young gerbils did not change as a result of PBN treatment.

An important animal model for studying senescence, developed in Japan, is the senescence-accelerated mouse. These mice develop conditions that are in many ways reminiscent of the human progerias described in Chapter 5, in that they display in an accelerated fashion many of the hallmarks of the normal aging process. Various substrains of this mouse have been developed, each displaying in isolation one or a few of the many deficits seen in the original strain. One of these substrains, called P8, ages normally in most of its body, but goes through age-dependent changes in the brain and in mental capacity in a greatly accelerated fashion. Functionally, P8 mice are similar to Alzheimer's patients, in that they undergo premature and aggressive degeneration of neurons, particularly pyramidal neurons in associative regions of the brain. This process is accompanied by the retraction and degradation of dendrites, a process usually seen only in old age. As in the normally aging brain, neuronal death results in a shrinkage of the brain tissues and in a loss of cognitive functions, especially learning and memory. Another substrain, P10, also shows a more Alzheimer's-like pathology, with premature accumulation of amyloid-filled neuritic plaques in the brain.

A possible involvement of oxidative damage in this process was recently examined by the same laboratory that carried out the gerbil studies just described. They found an accelerated increase in the accumulation of oxidatively damaged proteins, as well as membrane lipids, in the neurons of P8 mice. They also examined the effect of PBN on the development of disease in these mice. They found that administration of PBN over time reduced the accumulation of oxidative damage to both proteins and membranes in brain tissue. Experiments in other laboratories showed that antioxidants were able both to increase the lifespan of P8 mice and to significantly improve cognitive function.

If brain aging can be accelerated by oxidative damage, and this acceleration retarded by antioxidants, then it might be expected that caloric restriction, which is presumed to operate at least in part through a system-wide reduction in the generation of oxidative damage, should have a positive impact on brain damage and cognitive function as animals age. This has proved to be the case in a recent study in mice. As a measure of oxidation in aging brain cells, researchers again looked at the intracellular accumulation of oxidized proteins, this time in normal mice. Oxidatively damaged proteins were found to increase from eight through twenty-seven months of age, particularly in the hippocampus and other associative regions of the brain, in fully fed mice. Animals placed on a calorically restricted diet at weaning showed reductions of up to 50 percent in the amounts of intracellular oxidized protein; significant reductions were seen even when caloric restriction was started in adult mice. These researchers also compared the ability of fully fed and calorically restricted mice to learn and remember tasks as a function of age. In a shock-avoidance learning test, calorically restricted mice required only about half as many trials to learn how to avoid a mildly discomfiting shock as did age-matched fully fed controls. These results agree with earlier findings that calorically restricted animals show superior neurological function compared with fully fed animals.

In the end, the aging of the cells that make up the human brain turns out to be no different from the processes at work to guarantee the gradual post-reproductive decline of all the body's systems. A lessening of almost any of the brain's functions, whether coordination of our internal physiological systems or interpretation of our external environment, will gradually render us more susceptible to accidental death. Should that strategy fail, eventually senescence of the brain itself—as with any other major organ—will lead us to a "natural" death.

Yet undeniably, a gradual, drawn-out failure of the brain, with its accompanying collapse of mind, holds a particular fear. Heart attacks, stroke, or kidney failure, particularly when we are very old, will take us to the same certain fate, but it is something like Alzheimer's disease that we most dread. We would all like to go out in the end not just "with our boots on," but with a clear mind, an undistorted sense of who we are and what is happening to us. The enormous energy—and money—poured into research on Alzheimer's disease is a testament to our dread and to our need to understand both the normal and abnormal aging processes that can affect the mind. The fact that at bottom these processes prove to be nothing special should not worry us; we might have foreseen such a conclusion had we known more about aging in general before we became concerned about aging of the brain in particular.

But we do know more about aging now than ever before, thanks in large part to basic and clinical research funded by the National Institute of Aging. We have explored most of what is known in this and the preceding chapters. The question now before us is, what should we do with this information? Do we apply it simply to living longer, or should we concern ourselves with living better? Can we do both? These are the questions we will address in our final chapter.

11

A Conditional Benefit

In this book we have looked at the process of aging from a new and increasingly important perspective, that of cell and molecular biology and the underlying discipline of genetics. These are fairly new disciplines: Cell biology really came into its own only at the end of the last century; genetics was born in the first few years of the present century, with the rediscovery of Gregor Mendel's momentous works; and molecular biology emerged from the fields of biochemistry and microbial genetics only toward the end of the 1950s. These three disciplines have provided powerful new tools for looking at living organisms. We can now analyze biology at its most fundamental level; we can look for the genes underlying a given aspect of the life history of an animal, ask what exactly it is they do, how they do it, which other genes they may interact with, and how each gene's function may be affected by the environment. In the past twenty-five years or so, this new approach has been applied to the study of human physiology as well, and has given rise to an entirely new branch of medicine called molecular medicine. This new field will radically alter the way we approach diagnosing and treating human illness in the twenty-first century. But perhaps even more important than its impact on managing disease will be the new framework that molecular medicine provides for thinking about every aspect of human biology, including such perfectly normal processes as aging.

Genes, Senescence, and Death

There is every reason to believe that aging—senescence—is under genetic control. Senescence appeared at a specific point in evolution; all indications are that this was at the very earliest stages of eukaryotic evolution. Senescence and programmed death were already clearly present in early eukaryotes like paramecia. When unicellular life forms evolved into multicellular organisms, these genetic programs were maintained: Many of the very same senescence effector and senescence resistor genes can be found in paramecia, *C. elegans*, and humans. This high degree of conservation of the genes underlying senescence, across species so widely separated in evolutionary time, is one of the major arguments in favor of the early emergence of genes controlling senescence and compulsory death, as opposed to their gradual accumulation over evolutionary time. It is also convincing evidence in favor of strong selective pressures working to maintain their existence, in spite of apparently negative consequences for individuals bearing these genes. It is possible that a few senescence effector genes may have been incorporated randomly into the genomes of various species over time, but perhaps too little attention has been paid to the fact that senescence programs were already present and operating in the very earliest eukaryotes.

Another reason for believing that senescence is genetically controlled is that maximum lifespan is a species-specific, stably heritable attribute of the life history of the members of a species, which is essentially an a priori definition of a genetically controlled trait. This statement requires some qualification. In species where there is considerable heterogeneity in size—dogs, for example—there will also be a heterogeneity in maximum lifespan. Large breeds of dog have longer maximal lifespans than small breeds. But the point is that these lifespans are heritable within each breed. Most important of all, perhaps, it is the extremely close coordination of reproduction and senescence within the life history of different species, and the similarity of aging phenotypes in species with vastly different maximal lifespans, that point to the operation of an evolutionarily derived common set of genetically determined mechanisms underlying senescence.

Neither maximum lifespan nor senescence is a monogenic trait; there is no single gene that controls these parameters in even the biologically simplest species. We are only just beginning to perceive the molecular basis for senescence in cells, but enough information has been uncovered to provide us with a sense of how it all might work. A good deal of this information has been presented in the preceding chapters, but as is often the case, too much detail can obscure the larger picture, the sense of how it might all fit together. So let us try in this concluding chapter to understand at the organismal level exactly how individual genes might be responsible for aging.

What seems abundantly clear from experiments carried out in the past two decades is that far from being caused by randomly accruing, idiosyncratic collections of large numbers of different genes in each species, as suggested by current evolutionary theories of aging, a modest number of senescence effector genes and senescence resistor genes in eukaryotes are organized into a limited number of evolutionarily conserved senescence programs. The evolutionary origin of senescence as a process is almost certainly congruent with two events that appear to have happened very close in time, and very early in eukaryote evolution: the incorporation of oxygen-metabolizing prokaryotic cells as a means of dealing with the oxygen crisis, and the incorporation of sex into reproduction. Oxidative damage began in eukaryotes when they imported oxygen-utilizing bacteria and converted them into the energy-producing structures we now call mitochondria. These bacteria also brought along with them many of the genes for defense against oxidative damage, such as the antioxidant enzymes superoxide dismutase and catalase. Thus the basic components of programmed death— a set of senescence effector genes along with senescence resistor genes—may have been acquired by eukaryotes at the very beginning of their evolutionary existence. As with other senescence-related genes, all of these genes are hightly similar in virtually all eukaryotes.

Oxidative damage as an effector mechanism of senescence is extraordinarily potent, and must have been so from the very beginning; it probably did not require much further evolutionary refinement after the emergence of eukaryotes. Even now, life forms that die in a matter of weeks or months die from the very same underlying mechanisms as animals living fifty or a hundred years. Thus it is unlikely that much evolutionary energy has been spent generating senescence effector genes, or even senescence resistor genes. What has more likely occurred over evolutionary time is the accretion of senescence regulatory genes, controlling the exposure of eukaryotic organisms to greater or lesser risk, at earlier or later times in their life histories, from a relatively limited and evolutionary ancient number of senescence effector mechanisms. The target of senescence regulatory genes would likely be senescence repressor genes such as those for antioxidant enzymes or DNA repair systems. Senescence regulatory genes control the timing of onset of senescence; in so doing, they indirectly lengthen or shorten maximal lifespan. This could most easily be done by modulating the activity of senescence resistor genes.

We have discussed in previous chapters the specific functions of some of the genes involved in senescence, but it might be useful to think about just one gene and how it could participate in the overall senescence of an organism. An interesting example would be the gene responsible for Werner's syndrome (WS). It does not matter whether the Werner's gene turns out to be a true human aging gene or not—it certainly could, and probably will. The homolog of the Werner's gene in yeast definitely affects the aging process in those organisms. But for the moment we will simply use it as a general model for genes involved in cellular senescence and aging. Clearly, persons with WS exhibit many of the phenotypes of human aging. Given that normal aging is polygenic, while WS is a single-gene defect, it is not at all surprising that the overall syndrome is not perfectly congruent with the normal aging process.

The Werner's gene is now known to be a DNA helicase. To date, nine alleles have been identified for this gene that, when present in the same individual in two copies, can cause WS. Doubtless others will be uncovered as time goes on. How could a helicase be involved in cellular senescence? As we have said, senescence as a cellular process can be viewed as a balance between damage and repair. Damage to DNA is perhaps one of the most senescence-provoking types of damage a cell can experience, in both dividing and nondividing cells. A cell will do everything it can to repair this damage; if it fails to do so, the cell will either be shunted into a state of permanent senescence (the outcome of which is not entirely clear) or induced to undergo apoptosis.

Prior to reproductive maturity, DNA repair mechanisms are quite active, particularly in dividing cells, where DNA damage is more likely to arise in connection with DNA replication. DNA helicases play an important role in this process, because the DNA strands must be unwound before repair can begin. Helicases are often part of the various protein complexes that physically associate with DNA, maintaining the DNA in an appropriate state for carrying out functions such as replication, copying genes that are to be made into proteins, and repair of DNA damage. An altered function in any one of these proteins could contribute to cellular senescence, because each of these processes can be absolutely crucial to cellular function, but perhaps none is more crucial to cell survival than DNA repair. It is likely that there are a number of different helicase genes in our genomes, encoding helicases with different specific functions. The helicase unwinding DNA for purposes of replication may well be different from the helicase used for local DNA repair.

How could a defect in a DNA helicase gene result in the premature aging phenotypes seen in WS? Helicases would be among those genes we have classified as housekeeping genes, and so inherited alterations in their function could be expected to have an effect in essentially every cell in the body. We imagine this to be the basis for the widespread nature of the physiological changes seen in WS. If damage to DNA is accumulating at a normal rate in cells throughout the body, and repair of this damage is seriously compromised by a Werner's helicase allele, it is rather easy to imagine that these cells would experience accelerated senescence.

But how does this relate to normal aging? Can we make the stretch from involvement of a defective helicase gene in WS to the involvement of a normal helicase gene in the normal aging process? Reasonable scenarios are not all that difficult to envision. Let us imagine that at the time of reproductive maturation, perhaps under the influence of sex hormones, the activity of the normal helicase gene is turned down in all cells throughout the body. This will immediately affect each cell's ability to repair DNA. Each gene in the genome, in addition to containing the coding information for a protein, also has an associated

control region that is used to regulate the rate at which the corresponding protein is produced. These control regions respond to signals
sent throughout the body; hormones are a common example of such
signals. It is entirely conceivable that a turning down of the activity of
a repair helicase at sexual maturation is one part of a "program" of
senescence that will hasten the eventual death of an organism.

As we have seen, a diminution of DNA repair is in fact a normal
accompaniment of human aging; whether that happens as a result of
altered expression of a repair helicase, we cannot say. In persons
afflicted with WS, the helicase gene could be defective in a structural
sense, producing a protein with greatly decreased helicase function.
Alternatively, it may encode a normal helicase, but its control region
may be altered in such a way that abnormally low amounts of the protein are produced. In other words, the gene may operate *from birth* as
if the individual were sexually mature and ready for senescence to set
in. Either defect would explain the accelerated aging seen in Werner's
patients. Cells from Werner's patients do in fact show an unusually
high level of unrepaired DNA, including chromosomal abnormalities,
and damage of this type is thought to lead to either senescence or
death of the affected cells.

None of the foregoing is based on fact; it is entirely speculation.
Work is continuing on the helicase involved in WS, try to unravel its
role in this disease and the role of the corresponding normal helicase
in normal human aging. This will likely take a few years. The point of
the above exercise is to suggest how a defect in a single gene could lead
to expression of a wide range of aging-associated phenotypes. If a single gene could indeed cause the wide range of senescent phenotypes
seen in WS, it would reinforce the idea that aging may not necessarily
have to involve a huge number of genes. The estimate of seven to seventy genes, made by George Martin twenty years ago and dismissed
by some as far too low, seems increasingly reasonable. Whatever the
number, we imagine that the interaction of an individual's particular
combination of alleles for each of these genes, with each other and
with the environment, will determine that individual's unique rate and
path of senescence.

The Werner's gene, should it prove to be a true human senescence
effector gene, will also provide important lessons for our understanding of the evolution of senescence. First, it would show that a single

gene can have a powerful effect on the aging process. This would not be predicted by current theories of the evolution of senescence, which see aging as due to the gradual accumulation of large numbers of senescence-related genes over evolutionary time, each responsible for only a tiny portion of the aging process. A defect in only one of these genes would not be predicted to have such a large effect on aging. And the Werner's gene would join the growing list of genes that illustrate the tremendous evolutionary conservation of senescence effector genes. A gene in yeast has recently been shown to be the evolutionary ancestor of the Werner's gene, and it turns out to be involved in replicative senescence in these cells; disabling of this gene, called SGS1, causes an accelerated aging syndrome in yeast characterized by cellular defects similar to WS. And recall the human superoxide dismutase gene that was able to prolong lifespan in Drosophila. Current theories on the evolution of senescence do not predict that organisms widely separated in evolutionary time should have the same senescence-related genes; in fact, they predict the opposite.

One last word concerning the putative senescence regulator genes referred to in previous sections. We have postulated that reproductive hormones play a key role in regulating onset of the senescence program. Hormones tied to the reproductive cycle are clearly involved in one of the more spectacular examples we have of senescence in an animal. A very few animals, such as certain species of salmon, are semelparous—they reproduce only once, and then die very quickly thereafter. After several years of feeding in the open ocean, these salmon return to the rivers in which they originally hatched and make their way upstream to a suitable spawning ground. As soon as they enter the river, they stop feeding, relying on food they have stored while in the ocean to carry them through impressive hazards. The toll from accidental death during this journey is very high, and only a few survive to breed. Once breeding activities are finished, both sexes undergo extremely rapid physical deterioration, passing through the entire sequence of events leading to death in just a few days. Virtually every organ system in the body is involved. There is little question that initiation of this sequence is under genetic control, and that reproductive hormones play a major role in its mediation.

Yet it must be admitted that evidence bearing on the role of reproductive hormones as regulators of senescence in most animals is largely indirect. Senescence is greatly accelerated at the time of reproductive maturity. It is possible that there are separate sets of signals regulating reproductive maturity and the acceleration of senescence, but nature is not usually so wasteful. On the other hand, there is a good deal of evidence suggesting that senescence and reproductive hormones are intimately tied together, particularly in females. The life-prolonging effects of caloric restriction reflect a delayed onset of senescence, and this is accompanied by a delayed production of reproductive hormones in females. The growth of certain tumors is promoted by sex hormones, which would certainly hasten senescence and death. Sex hormones are important in the development of the reproductive system in the early years, but both their production and the tissues affected by them change dramatically in the reproductive years and, especially in female mammals, in the post-reproductive years.

In humans, cardiovascular disease is clearly a major idiopathic component of senescence in humans. At menopause, when estrogen stops being produced internally, the rate of cardiovascular disease, which is low in premenopausal women, climbs rapidly to the level observed in men. On the other hand, post-menopausal women receiving estrogen (a sex hormone) replacement therapy have a greatly reduced incidence of heart disease. It has recently been shown that estrogen administration also reduces the incidence of Alzheimer's disease—another major senescence-induced disease—by nearly 50 percent in post-menopausal women. The same is true for osteoporosis and a variety of other senescence-related disorders. In the absence of any evidence to the contrary, and in the presence of a great deal of indirect supporting evidence, it seems reasonable to assume that reproductive hormones are the most likely regulators of senescence in humans, and in fact probably in the majority of multicellular animals with reproductive hormone systems.

With completion of the Human Genome Project early in the next century, it is entirely possible that one day we will actually know the identity of all of the genes involved in aging, the types of alleles of these genes spread among the population, and to a first approximation, how they work. What will we do with this information? We will certainly want to use it to increase the quality of human life, particularly toward the end of our years when the cumulative ravages of senescence cause the most suffering. But can we, will we in the course of this quest, also increase the quantity of human life? Can we live longer?

Scientific disclaimers notwithstanding, this question probably drives a significant proportion of all gerontological research. It can be approached in two different ways. The first approach, which is of immediate interest to most of us, is to ask this question in terms of average lifespan: How long, on average, can we expect to live, and what, if anything, can we do to increase this expectation? Average lifespan in human populations is determined by two things and, as far as we know, only two things: the rate of accidental death and the rate of death driven by senescence (including accidents caused indirectly by senescence). The second approach to the question of longevity addresses a more fundamental biological question, namely, that of human maximum possible lifespan. We would very much like to know whether there are any fundamental biological determinants underlying human maximum lifespan, and whether and to what extent these may be mutable. Let us begin with this question first.

Maximum Human Lifespan

When we compare the endpoints of curves C and D in Figure 1.1, the implied maximum lifespan for humans born in the nineteenth and twentieth centuries does not seem to be terribly different. Of course, the numbers of people surviving to the most advanced ages is small, making any meaningful comparisons statistically suspect. And certainly, a single century in the evolutionary lifetime of a species that reproduces as slowly as humans is less than the blink of an eye. Still, the historical record, as far as we can determine, supports the idea that maximum human lifespan may not have changed at all in the past 5000 years or so. While still a brief period in evolutionary terms, an apparent constancy of human maximal lifespan over 5000 years at least raises the question of whether this is a mutable factor in the life history of human beings.

As we continue to rectangularize the human survival curve shown in Figure 1.1C, through medical and social interventions, average lifespan will continue to increase. But there is an implied limit to this increase; as such curves approach perfect rectangularity, average human lifespan will approach the inherent theoretical maximum. Based on current projections of the increase in average human lifespan (Table 11.1), and the difference in survival between males and females, we

Table 11.1. *Expected age at death for persons born in the years 2000 and 2050, and for those turning 65 in the years 2000 and 2050*

	Caucasian		Black		Hispanic	
	B[a]	65[b]	B[a]	65[b]	B[a]	65[b]
2000						
Males	74.2	81.2	64.6	78.8	75.2	83.1
Females	80.5	84.7	74.7	82.9	82.8	87.4
2050						
Males	82.0	86.6	70.8	81.5	84.4	90.6
Females	85.9	88.6	79.7	85.3	89.6	92.9

[a] Expected age of death at birth.

[b] Expected age at death for someone 65 years of age.

Source: Middle assumption data taken from U.S. Bureau of the Census life expectancy tables, July 1993.

could guess that women born somewhere in the twenty-sixth century will have come very close to this apparent limit. What happens then? Based on what we think we understand about the basic biology of aging, will it ever be possible to move the entire rectangle itself to the right; can we increase maximum possible human lifespan?

Before trying to answer that question, let's take a look at what maximum human lifespan is currently thought to be. We could approach this question intuitively and anecdotally—simply find the longest person that ever lived, and that must be the maximum possible human lifespan, or very close to it. The problem is that anecdotal information is notoriously unreliable. Those who study this question closely regard almost every claim for human age beyond 110 or so with great skepticism. Independent records for the vast majority of such claims do not exist, and people over 100 years of age almost always have serious problems with memory. Many claims are knowingly false, made to improve social standing or attract fame. In seventeenth-century England, one Thomas Parr claimed an age of 150, and was buried with appropriate honors in Westminster Abbey at the supposed age of 152. An autopsy on Parr's remains was carried out by no less a figure than William Harvey, who found his organs suspiciously young in appearance. Parr is now believed to have been no more than ninety when he died. It was long accepted that a high proportion of individuals in the Caucasus region of what is now the Georgian Republic lived routinely beyond 120 or even 130 years. However, upon even moderately close inspection, virtually every such claim has either been dropped for lack of evidence or shown to be an outright fraud.

The oldest human being whose age can be absolutely verified was Jeanne Louise Calment, born February 21, 1875. Mme. Calment lived in her native city of Arles, France, until her death at the age of 122 years and nearly six months on August 4, 1997. Although blind and nearly deaf, she was nonetheless alert mentally until the very end. She served as a living memory source for her community; as a teenager, she sold paint in her father's shop to Vincent Van Gogh, who spent a year in Arles in 1888. Mme. Calment's long life paid off in many ways. In 1965, at the age of ninety, she entered into an agreement with an attorney to sell him her apartment *en viager*; he agreed to pay her $500 a month for as long as she lived, which would entitle him to inherit her apartment upon her death. Given her already advanced age, it probably seemed a shrewd piece of business on his part. The attorney died in 1995, after having paid her more than twice the market value of her apartment. His survivors inherited the burden of his promissary note and continued making payments to Mme. Calment until her death nearly three years later.

So at present, at the level of verification of a single individual's documentable age, we can say with some confidence that *absolute* human lifespan is at least 122 and a half years. But that doesn't mean that someone in the past has not actually exceeded that age; we would have no way of knowing one way or the other. And as more and more people live past 100 years, exceeding Mme. Calment's age is certainly possible, and perhaps likely. The oldest person alive at the time of this writing, whose age is beyond dispute (among demographers, as opposed to the Guiness Book of Records), is Chris Mortensen, a San Rafael, California, man who turned 115 years of age just four days after Mme. Calment died. Studies with fruit flies have shown clearly that when very large numbers of very old individuals are observed, previously unimaginable survival ages are uncovered. The same will almost certainly be true of humans. But will these numbers represent a fundamental shift of the entire curve to the right, or will they simply be an elongation of the flattened-out tail-end of the human survival curve (Fig. 1.1C, D)? The latter seems the most likely interpretation.

Even with human populations of the size used in the very best demographic analyses of the endpoint of human life, the number of people who are "pushing the envelope" of human age (i.e., are over 110) is at any given time rarely more than fifty in all of the countries for which we have reliable data. With such small numbers, it is simply not possible to decide statistically what the maximum lifespan for human beings is, and statistics is the language of demography. So a definition of maximum lifespan remains as elusive as the position of an electron in its orbit around a nucleus, and it is defined in essentially the same way. No demographer concerned about his or her professional credibility would ever specify a number. However, in a roomful of demographers, it might be possible (if they thought none of their colleagues were listening too closely) to get about half of them to agree that *statistically* the number *appears* to lie somewhere between 110 and 120 years at the present time.

Since demographers will not commit themselves on whether maximum lifespan even exists, let alone whether it could be a mutable value, we must turn once again to basic biology and ask whether anything we have uncovered in gerontological research over the past fifty years or so would convince us that maximal human lifespan can be extended. One obvious focus for a discussion of the plasticity of maximum lifespan is caloric restriction (Chapter 8). In every caloric restriction study that has been carried out, the measurable maximum lifespan of warm-blooded animals has been increased by restricting their caloric intake. The animals subjected to such regimens are healthier and show less signs of aging at every point in their calendrically measured lives. We are not talking about simply a shift of average lifespan to the right, although this also occurs. These studies involve large numbers of animals, followed from birth to death with very tight record-keeping; it is beyond question that maximal lifespan, by any and all measures, has been increased.

Nevertheless, many scientists are uncertain of just what this means. Every experiment needs controls for proper interpretation of data. The controls in the caloric restriction experiments have traditionally been considered to be the fully fed animals. Great care has always been

taken to match vital dietary components such as vitamins and minerals and other trace elements between calorically restricted and fully fed
controls. The problem lies in deciding which group is really the experimental group, and which is the control. It has been argued that the
animals subjected to caloric restriction are dietarily much closer to life
in the wild than are those reared on an unlimited food supply. The
point can certainly be made that the real experimental animals in these
studies have been those subjected to the artificially calorie-rich diets
provided in a protected laboratory environment under conditions of
minimal physical exercise.

What we have learned from these experiments may well be that
excess caloric intake shortens maximal lifespan, not that caloric restriction extends it. From that point of view, the data on true maximum
human lifespan is probably already there, in developing countries
where caloric intake is considerably below that in more industrialized
societies. Unfortunately, other factors affecting human survival are
often less than optimal in these countries, limiting the number of people who would approach the theoretical limit of human life. Together
with a lack of reliable records, and the fact that very likely caloric
intake will go up in these countries as their economic situation
improves, there seems little likelihood of deriving the needed information from this source.

While the caloric restriction experiments do not convince us that
they can contribute much to increasing the actual human maximum
lifespan, they nevertheless leave open the possibility that we may not
currently be realizing the full *potential* maximum lifespan for humans,
and that this may well be within our reach. Although meaningful data
on larger animals have not yet been gathered, the limited amount of
evidence we do have at present suggests that the results of caloric
restriction seen in experiments with rats and mice would likely be true
for the higher primates, including humans. Some of the rigors of
caloric restriction in humans could possibly be reduced with the aid of
appetite suppressants such as the natural protein product leptin, which
has proved incredibly effective in animal studies. There are of course
problems in extrapolating both the methodology and the anticipated
results from caloric restriction experiments in rodents to humans:
What caloric baseline should we devise for humans? How far below
this baseline should we go? When in life should caloric restriction be

started in humans? How will individuals balance caloric restriction with perceived quality of life? These questions are not easy to answer. But we can hazard the guess that if adult humans in most Western countries *on average* restricted their caloric intake by 20 to 25 percent, in the context of present-day standards of life-style and health care, we could reasonably expect to see an increase in average lifespan, and we might possibly see an increase in apparent maximum lifespan as well.

But to the extent that true maximum lifespan is a genetically controlled characteristic, it follows that it will change only on an evolutionary time scale, which under normal circumstances is so far beyond the lifespan of individuals and even societies that it becomes an essentially immutable number. Of course, circumstances are not always normal. Cataclysmic events can greatly accelerate evolution; the apparent impact of a major meteorite on the earth sixty million years ago caused a rapid, highly compressed burst of evolutionary change. In a sense, the experiments we discussed in Chapter 3 involved a form of evolutionary cataclysm. In one experiment, the researchers selected eggs only from the oldest females for propagation; from an evolutionary perspective, they were "killing off" flies from eggs laid early in a female's lifespan. The result was a fairly rapid shift in average and maximal lifespans. The same effect was achieved by exposing guppies to predators targeting pre-versus post-reproductive guppies. And it seems safe to say that overfeeding can very quickly reduce maximum lifespan. So although genetically controlled, maximum lifespan is not immutable, it can change in response to changes in the environment; the speed at which it changes will depend on the rate and extent of environmental change.

But clearly there is a genetic element in maximum lifespan, and as far as we understand at present this is largely a reflection of genetic control of the timing of reproduction, for it is only with the onset of reproduction that the pace of senescence sets in with full force. The present reproductive pattern in humans is something we neither know how to change nor would want to change even if we could. This is a pattern that evolved over, at a minimum, hundreds of thousands of years, in response to the forces of natural selection, in individuals living in the wild. It is not obvious that these conditions are even relevant to further human development; human reproductive patterns may well now be governed as much or more by cultural factors as by environmental conditions.

The bottom line is that everything we know about maximum possible lifespan in animals generally, and about evolution, suggests that true human maximal lifespan will not likely change in the absence of some sort of natural or man-made disaster. Aside from changing our dietary habits to avoid an unnatural foreshortening of our natural lifespan, the kinds of changes that would be required to perturb true human maximal lifespan are probably unacceptable. This leads us to the speculation that as some of the current major causes of senescence and death in humans, such as cardiovascular disease and cancer, are brought under control, other manifestations of senescence will move forward to take their place. Alzheimer's disease is just one such example; there may be many more that we are barely aware of at the present time. The most likely projection is that as senescence-related disease causes of death are gradually eliminated, we will see nature's backup plan in its final form; average lifespan will increase at the population level, but as individuals, our major organ systems will gradually grow weaker until we simply expire. More and more death certificates will read "died of natural causes." This is not a bad goal in itself.

Average Human Lifespan

Unlike the situation with maximum lifespan, the outlook for *average* human lifespan—what demographers often refer to as life expectancy—is much more hopeful. There is no question that average lifespan is presently on the rise throughout most of the world; the rate of increase in industrialized countries has been nothing less than spectacular in this century (Fig. 11.1), and is slowly but steadily increasing in other parts of the world as well. The most important factors in this increase have been improved public health measures and personal hygiene, lifestyle changes affecting health, and improved medical care, probably in that order. Widespread immunization, reductions in the incidence and severity of physical trauma, improvements in diet, the development of antibiotics, decreased mortality for women and infants at childbirth and for post-menopausal women—the impact of all of these on human survival are well known to epidemiologists and

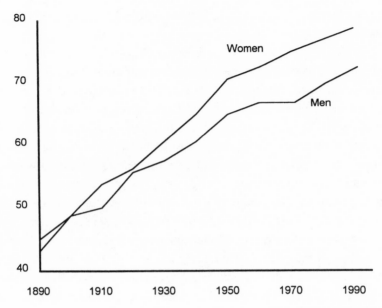

Figure 11.1. Changes in average lifespan in the United States over the past 100 years.

demographers. All of these changes affect the shape of the curve shown in Figure 1.1C, leading to its "rectangularization" and pulling the average human lifespan ever higher. The only serious countervailing trend during this period stems from the effects of widespread smoking, particularly among men, but that may at last be diminishing somewhat in a few Western countries. There have been periodic countervailing trends in some populations associated with catastrophic events such as wars and, even into this century, major plagues caused by infectious disease. But the overall direction of average lifespan in this century has been one of steady increase.

Average human lifespan is clearly determined by both genetics and the environment. The environmental impact on average lifespan involves various forms of accidental death: infectious diseases, accidents, and lifestyle choices—smoking, for example. The gains in lifespan shown in Figure 11.1 are due almost entirely to controlling accidental causes of death. A genetic influence on average lifespan is revealed by things such as the identical twins study, which showed that identical twins have average lifespans much closer to one another than do fraternal twins. It has also been observed that individuals who live to very old ages tend to have offspring that also survive to older ages than the population as a whole. Average lifespan will reflect variations among individuals in the genetic control of the basic processes of senescence itself and the resulting occurrence of idiopathic diseases such as cancer, diabetes, and heart disease. Control of senescence-related causes of death has made very little contribution to the gains shown in Figure 11.1. However, as accidental causes of death are increasingly brought under control, additional gains in average lifespan will be increasingly dependent on our ability to affect senescence-induced diseases. Of course, we will never be able to control true physical accidents—falling off a cliff, drowning, being hit by a car. But as the average lifespan of persons not dying by these means pulls ever closer to the limit of true maximal lifespan, additional gains will come almost entirely from our ability to influence the fundamental mechanisms of senescence.

Before we launch into a discussion of the possibilities of further increases in average human lifespan, let's reflect for a moment on just what we would hope to accomplish by such an increase. At a population level, any increase in the average lifespan value will look good on demographic charts. But how do we want to move the average value upward? If it is simply a matter of adding years to the ends of our lives, would this necessarily be a good thing? The end years of our lives are not always the best years, characterized by increasing failure of most of our physical and mental faculties. As we look at many of the oldest old in our own families and in our communities, we must ask ourselves whether simply adding another five years or so to the end of their lives would be in anyone's best interest. In many cases we could probably say yes, but for those suffering from senescence-related diseases and disabilities, for those already exhausted by the ravages of old age, we—and the aged individuals themselves—might well say no. Almost everyone would agree that what we would really like to do is extend the middle years of life, when we are still vigorous and able to experience life at its fullest. We will of course want to continue exploring ways of easing the travails of the end years of our lives, but where we might profit most from adding more years is somewhere in the middle.

Tracking increases in average human lifespan is a relatively straightforward task that, at least in some parts of the world, can be carried out with considerable precision. For human populations, the first requirement for good demographic studies relating to lifespan (especially as it affects the oldest old) is unimpeachable, government-maintained birth and death records going back a minimum of a hundred years. Only a handful of countries have such records. The United States is not one of them; birth and death records have traditionally been the responsibility of individual states, and the information gathered and its method of reporting and verification have varied widely. Only with the advent of the Social Security system in the 1930s, and the Medicare system in the 1960s, did the United States begin to have a national, standardized system for birth, death, and age verification comparable to most European countries. Thus one of the populations that many demographers would like to know the most about is often excluded from larger studies of aging because of the unreliability of all but the most recent data. However, the twenty or so countries with a longer tradition of accurate national birth and death statistics have a combined population approximating that of the United States—over 300 million people—which provides a reasonable data base for longer-range demographic analysis.

One of the more remarkable facts to emerge from detailed analyses of maximum lifespan is that the mortality rate—the number of individuals dying per year at any given age per 1000 persons of that age in the population—has been dropping dramatically over the past fifty years for the oldest old and for centenarians. The data shown in Fig. 11.2 were compiled from the registries of those European countries (plus Japan) that have the longest and most accurate birth/death record-keeping systems. All indications are that exactly the same trend is under way in the United States. The rate at which both men and women are dying in these two age categories has been dropping at a rate of 5 percent or more per decade since 1950, and there is no sign that it is leveling off. One obvious result of this trend is that the percentage of elderly people in all industrialized countries has just about doubled in the past thirty years (Table 11.2). In the eighty- to ninety-nine-year-old age group, the trend toward lower mortality is more pronounced in women than in men. This is not a statistical fluke; it is true of every single country for which reliable data can be gathered, including the United States. (The apparently similar gender differential in the decline among centenarians is not considered statistically significant, due to the small numbers involved.)

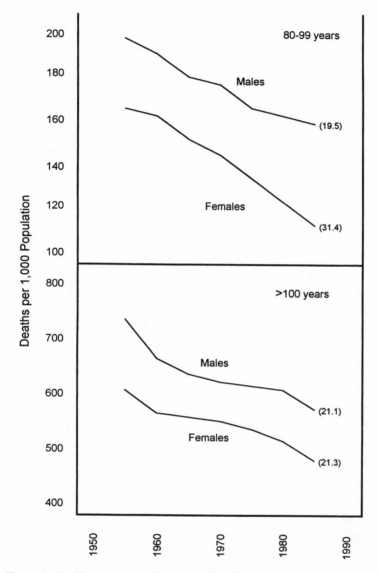

Figure 11.2. Changing mortality among the oldest old and centenarians.

The reasons for the decline in mortality rates among the oldest people in society over the past fifty years are not particularly mysterious. The same factors that have acted to increase average longevity have in this century also produced increasing numbers of people surviving to the ages that are the starting point for surveys of the oldest old. Peo-

Table 11.2. *Persons over 80 as a percentage of the total population in countries with the best birth/death registries*

Country	1960	1980
Austria	1.7	3.6
England/Wales	1.9	3.7
France	2.0	3.7
Italy	1.6	3.0
Holland	1.3	2.9
Japan	0.7	2.3
Sweden	1.8	4.2
Switzerland	1.5	3.6
Average	1.6	3.4

ple in general are taking better care of themselves and are being better cared for by society, and this is played out in terms of longer life. Assuming that age at death reflects a stochastic process, simply increasing the number of old people in itself is bound to generate points farther out along the age axis at which some people will die. Individuals surviving beyond ninety years or so are also likely to be more genetically "fit," in the sense that they were less susceptible to conditions such as cancer or heart disease that are responsible for death at an earlier age in the majority of humans. As more people survive into their hundreds, we can expect to pick up more "outliers" along the age axis, but as stated earlier, this would not in itself necessarily signal a change in true human maximum lifespan.

But what about the rest of us, who may not have inherited a set of genes propelling us into the heady ranks of the very oldest old? Can we expect that the average survival age will continue to increase, and the mortality rate decrease, in the years ahead? Insurance companies and the Social Security Administration are betting on it. Predictions are always risky; we do not yet know, for example, just what effect the AIDS epidemic will have on average human lifespan long-term, particularly if the virus causing it should mutate to a more infectious form. If not turned aside in the relatively near future, we may see an infectious organism's impact on human survival for the first time in nearly a hundred years.

Nevertheless, average lifespans for the U.S. population as a whole are expected to continue increasing at a rate of between 0.8 and 1 percent per decade between the years 2000 and 2050. These projections are based largely on assumptions about the generation of new knowledge relating to human genetics and physiology, about the rapid translation of this knowledge into useful medical procedures by the private sector and by physicians, and finally, and perhaps most important, about the dissemination of this knowledge to the general public, especially where this knowledge can be used to guide personal choices concerning health care and lifestyle. The rate of increase in longevity projected for the first part of the twenty-first century is considerably lower than that experienced in the first half of the twentieth century (Fig. 11.1). Between 1900 and 1950, average lifespan in the United States increased at a rate of about 7 percent per decade; in the second half of the century, this rate fell to about 3 percent per decade. We can expect that the overall rate of increase in longevity will continue to decline as we continue to control the causes of accidental death and as the more difficult to control senescence-related causes of death continue to move to the fore.

But at What Cost?

We have more than enough information in hand, and it is sufficiently underutilized at present, that we may be confident that average human lifespan will continue to increase for some time to come. The increases will not continue at the pace seen in the twentieth century, because most accidental disease causes of death have been brought under control. As average lifespan moves ever closer to the theoretical maximum, the rate of gain will be inexorably slow. But it is abundantly clear that all of the things touted in recent years by health experts for increasing the quality of human life—a moderate diet, rich in fresh fruits and vegetables; reasonable levels of exercise; avoidance of excessive chemical toxins, including those in cigarette smoke, alcohol, and recreational drugs—will also increase the quantity of human life. And they will do so by adding years to the middle of our lives, when we are most active and productive, and not just to the end of our lives, when we are often feeble and suffering. Together with continued research into means for controlling senescence-related diseases and disabilities in these end years or, at the very least, lessening the physical discomfort and the mental anguish that accompany them, there is enormous potential for increasing both the quality and the quantity of human life. Just as we may well not be reaching our maximal lifespan as individuals at present, we are almost certainly not realizing as a species our potential average lifespan, and for largely overlapping reasons.

As we race toward the new millennium, and increasingly avail ourselves of the information and technologies to achieve longer and more productive lives, we must never forget that if we succeed there will be underlying costs, and that these are potentially heavy costs. As we continue to improve the health of persons in what we might call the "youngest-old" category—fifty to sixty-five years—we will unquestionably increase the number of people surviving into the old, oldest-old, and centenarian age groups. For many of our elderly, these are "high maintenance" years. The incidence of chronic, debilitating idiopathic diseases such as Alzheimer's disease, stroke, Parkinson's disease, and many others increases almost exponentially past age eighty-five or so. The care of human beings with these disorders is enormously expensive. Most such individuals are completely unable to sustain themselves, either on a personal level or financially, in terms of monies they may have set aside to provide for their later years. Ideally, we should wait until these diseases are under control before producing more people who are almost certain to get them, but that is unlikely to happen.

The problem does not go away simply by finding cures for these diseases. The cost/benefit ratios of eliminating diseases are usually calculated in terms of the investment necessary to cure a disease versus the resulting savings in the cost of having to treat the disease, a reduction in the number of work days lost, the cost of supporting families during the illness of wage earners, and other economic factors, somehow all merged together with perceived increases in the quality of life. In other words, these considerations are usually focussed on individuals in the early and middle years of their lives. However, when elimination of a disease primarily increases the quantity of life in the years after an individual stops working, an additional economic factor is created: the cost of maintaining that now-healthy individual through Social Security or private pension funds. Fairly simple calculations can show that elimination of either heart disease or cancer would result in an enormous burden on the Social Security system as it is presently structured, in terms of the additional person-years of financial support required to maintain the survivors.

Yet we can be almost certain that the toll taken on our population by these two diseases alone will continue to diminish as a result of current investments in biomedical research. No one would want to reverse the trend toward conquering these diseases, but neither private nor public retirement systems are presently equipped to handle the added years of retirement their elimination would generate. Social Security, Medicare, and Medicaid benefits already account for more than one-third of all federal spending in the United States. By some estimates, Social Security will be paying out more than it takes in by the year 2012, and the Medicare Hospital Insurance trust fund will be depleted by the year 2001. How much more can the system absorb?

Currently, about 15 percent of persons over seventy years of age require some sort of assistance in their daily lives. This figure is likely to increase, perhaps substantially, before biomedical research into the diseases of the elderly is able to bring it down. Families of these people, in addition to having to deal with the emotional stress of caring for their loved ones, will be increasingly hard-pressed financially to bear the costs of supporting them. In the coming decades we will likely see more in the United States of what is currently happening in Japan—children of the oldest-old will themselves be retired and unable to assume even a modest portion of the costs of maintaining their parents. Increasingly, we can expect that these costs will be borne by society at large through Medicare and other social support programs. That is perhaps as it should be, but the money to do so will have to come from somewhere. It will come from those in society still able to work.

This could not have come at a worse time, because the proportion of the population that works in all countries throughout the world is dropping precipitously. Until very recently, demographers were concerned about a rapidly increasing human population crowding itself and everything else off the planet. No longer. The latest United Nations report on population shows that birth rates have fallen off dramatically all over the world in recent years. A birth rate of 2.1 children per woman per lifetime is currently required in Western countries to maintain the population at a steady level—the so-called "replacement level" of fertility. (The extra 0.1 child is necessary to make up for the children lost through accidental death prior to their own reproductive period.) The birth rate in the United States has been below 2.0 per woman for the past quarter-century. The birth rate in the industrialized countries as a whole is currently about 1.6 per woman per lifetime. In underdeveloped countries, the rate has fallen from six just thirty years ago to less than three today. Somewhere around 2040, if this trend continues, the birth rate in the world as a whole will be just about at the population replacement level, which means no additional population growth. World population would likely peak at about nine billion persons, and then possibly begin to fall.

Thus it is clear that as we increase the health and physical well-being of persons in the youngest-old age range, we will have to ask them—we will have to ask *ourselves*—to work longer, to direct more income into either public or private health care maintenance and retirement pension systems, and to think of retirement from work at age seventy or seventy-five, rather than sixty-five. This in itself is not unreasonable; if we are strong and healthy during these years, then remaining active, contributing to our communities and society at large, will enrich and very likely prolong our lives even further. But we must begin planning for this now. The current efforts by the U.S. Congress to restructure the Social Security and Medicare systems are founded on precisely the concerns just described. If we do not change them, these systems will simply become bankrupt. All of us need to become involved in discussions of these issues, both at work and in our communities. We must understand that if we are to live longer, there will have to be changes in the way our working and retirement years are structured.

Unfortunately, discussion of these issues will be complicated by the fact that precise predictions of key factors, such as the actual rate of increase in longevity over the coming decades, the timing of the availability of cures for age-related diseases, and the cost of maintaining the oldest-old versus old patients (the former may well be less expensive) are simply not available at present. This will allow some political leaders to downplay the seriousness of these issues, and their potential costs, on the assumption that that is what we want to hear. We must not let them do that; if we begin planning now on the basis of worst-case, or at least average-case assumptions, it will always be possible to back away later and redirect any monies over-committed to caring for the elderly in other directions. On the other hand, if we underestimate the seriousness of the problem now and fail to take the necessary steps soon, it may be extremely painful to play catch-up at a later date.

The resulting shift in the balance of age groups in our society caused by a combination of increased longevity and reduced birth rates will certainly have profound political as well as demographic implications. We have seen in recent years the increasing political power of well-organized collectives of senior citizens who, after all, have a lifetime of experience in dealing with the world at every level, including the political. This trend will only continue for the foreseeable future, and their newfound power may well come to be resented by other segments of society. Younger age groups are not likely to enjoy hearing that they will have to work beyond the age in life when their parents and grandparents retired. They will doubtless not be happy to hear that their Social Security taxes will be raised to support the increasing numbers of elderly, even though they will themselves one day benefit from this same support structure. But someone will have to deliver this message, and soon.

Finally, of course, we must bear in mind that all of these changes will not occur in a geopolitical vacuum, and that longevity will not increase throughout the world at the same pace. We can be sure that an underdeveloped country, barely able to feed itself and with an average lifespan of fifty years or so, will view the problem of caring for centenarians with little sense of urgency. Perhaps even more critical may be events already unfolding in developing countries. With increasingly effective public health and vaccination programs, and effective distribution systems for antibiotics and other medicines, these countries are starting to experience the rapid increases in longevity seen in the West in the early and middle parts of the twentieth century. Life expectancy in these so-called "second-world" countries has risen from about forty years in 1950 to about sixty-three years today. While the economies of these countries, with international help, have been able to support the public health programs that have led to these changes, they do not have the means—and there is no international agency to help them—to deal with the burgeoning numbers of older citizens that have resulted. The health care systems of these countries are caught in a dilemma: They must continue fighting to eradicate the infectious diseases that still ravage some of the younger members of their societies, while at the same time they struggle to deal with the chronic idiopathic diseases afflicting their new elderly members. Most have not yet developed social security programs to deal with simple maintenance of elderly populations, let alone come to grips with their highly specialized medical needs. Meanwhile, these countries, too, are beginning to experience significant declines in birthrate, which means the economic base for supporting social programs is eroding just at the time it is most critically needed.

So what seems like a rather simple and uncomplicated aim—the desire to live a longer, healthier, fuller life—turns out to have enormous ramifications, because it entails far-reaching demographic, social, and political changes. But we will rise to the occasion, as we always have in the past. As we continue to unravel the genetic basis of senescence and aging, we will continue to rectangularize the human survival curve; we may even move the entire curve slightly to the right, closer to its theoretical "true" value. Average human lifespan will continue to increase, and this will force changes upon us as a society. But these changes could hardly be more momentous than those we have passed through in the century that is about to end. A major part of the impetus for creating social security systems in the first place, in this and other countries, was the revolution in public health and medical care that resulted in increasing numbers of people surviving into old age. So we did it— we created the systems and institutions we needed, in spite of the hand-wringers of the time. If we need to restructure them, we will do that, too, and create new ones if we have to.

What Lies Ahead?

We have made an enormous investment in aging research over the past several decades, and the payoff has been an unprecedented insight into the basic mechanisms of aging. Such knowledge is absolutely essential if we are to lessen the burden of aging to us as individuals, as families, and as a society. We need to know the limits of what we can do, but we also want to know the full range of possibilities for extending and improving human life. So what are some of the insights yet to be gained, and where will they come from?

We have discussed the notion that the aging of cells, which underlies the aging of individuals, reflects an increasing burden of unrepaired damage to our DNA. If that is true, what will we see in Dolly, the sheep that gained fame in 1997 as the first truly cloned mammal? Dolly was cloned by removing the nucleus from a mammary gland cell taken from a six-year-old sheep. That nucleus was implanted into an unfertilized egg from another sheep, and proceeded to direct successfully the construction of an entire new sheep—Dolly. If we believe that the age of an animal is a reflection of the aging of its DNA, what age is Dolly? The nuclear DNA that directed her complete development was six years old. Does Dolly begin life at age six, in terms of cumulative DNA damage? Will she die prematurely from a form of artificially created progeria?

The story is even slightly more complex. There are two kinds of DNA in cells—nuclear and mitochondrial DNA. Damage to mitochondrial DNA is thought to be very important in the aging of cells. But inheritance of mitochondrial DNA is different from the inheritance of nuclear DNA. Mitochondrial DNA comes only from the mother, as part of her egg; sperm contribute no mitochondria to the newly formed individual. So Dolly has old nuclear DNA and fresh, new mitochondrial DNA from the egg into which the old nucleus was implanted. Which DNA will determine her age? Or will the nuclear DNA be somehow "rejuvenated" by the fresh egg, making her birth age and age in terms of cellular senescence the same? These are intriguing questions, the answers to which will have important implications for both ends of life: embryonic development and old age.

We will also want to follow the telomerase story closely as it unfolds in the next few years. There will doubtless be advantages to the ability to reactivate telomerase in cells that ordinarily do not divide. A commonly cited example is in the case of burn victims. The best skin for transplanting onto burns is the victim's own skin, and in the case of small burns this is entirely feasible and works well. In the case of massive burns, the victim simply doesn't have enough skin, and is too fragile to compromise by further skin removal. There have been attempts to grow some of an individual's skin cells in vitro for reimplantation to a burn site, but this has not been terribly successful because of the slow and ultimately limited growth potential of normal skin cells in culture. If telomerase were reactivated in some of these cells, we could well see the very rapid growth of sufficient cells to provide clinically useful amounts of a patient's own skin. The problem, of course, is how to stop the cells from continuing to grow once the burn site has been completely filled in. This is not beyond technical possibility, but great care would have to be taken to assure that skin cancer did not develop.

Whether the ability to control the expression of telomerase will ever have an impact on human aging is much more problematic. The danger in removing one of the body's major barriers to cancer is self-evident. But beyond that, we must remember that the majority of cells in the body do not divide, and for those cells replicative senescence is not a likely cause of aging. It is not at all obvious at present that reactivating telomerase in those cells would have any impact on aging of the tissues they make up. But this must be explored, nevertheless; current views could be wrong, in ways we cannot yet perceive. Could we rejuvenate those cells in our bodies that do divide by reactivating telomerase? It may be possible, through some form of gene therapy, which we will describe in a moment. But even if we could achieve that, aging in our other tissues—if it proves not to involve telomerase—would proceed on schedule, and it is not clear that our overall rate of aging would be seriously altered. Nevertheless, the importance of the ability to manipulate a major component of cellular senescence cannot be overstated, and we will all want to follow this story closely.

One of the largest sources of new information about human biology generally in the coming years will be the Human Genome Project. Scheduled for completion early in the twenty-first century, the Genome Project will provide us for the first time with a complete catalog—the precise DNA sequences—of all of the estimated 100,000 genes in the human genome. Of most immediate interest to the new breed of "molecular physicians" will be the genes responsible for the approximately 4000 heritable genetic diseases—a number of which have already been isolated and cloned. But we can also expect to find and ultimately identify the genes involved with the fundamental processes of cellular senescence. Some of these, too, have already been identified, including those disposing toward certain forms of senescence-related diseases such as cancer, Alzheimer's disease, and cardiovascular disease, as well as genes like p53, Rb, and telomerase.

One potential application of this new information is in gene therapy, wherein inherited defective copies of genes can be supplemented with good gene copies produced in the laboratory, using the blueprint provided by the Genome Project. The end products of all genes are the myriad proteins used by cells to carry on their daily functions. In some cases, particularly where the protein is used primarily outside of the cell producing it (hormones, for example), good copies of the defective protein can be administered to the body directly. But for most proteins made and utilized within the cell itself, this approach usually will not work. In gene therapy as it is currently being practiced, a good copy of a gene is incorporated into an appropriate "vector," usually some form of altered virus, for delivery to those cells most critically affected by the genetic defect. Once inside the targeted cell, the new genes make their way into the nucleus, where they are read by the cell's machinery just as if they were part of the cell's own DNA, and the cell is then able to make functional copies of the needed protein. Clinical trials for this form of "restorative" gene therapy are currently under way for nearly a dozen inherited human diseases, with many more in advanced planning stages.

In one sense, the immediate impact on aging of gene therapy may seem likely to be relatively minor, since of the genetic disorders currently targeted for treatment (certain cancers and cardiovascular disorders aside) few are directly involved with senescence and aging. Moreover, one of the major differences between aging and the genetic diseases currently being treated by gene therapy is that the latter are all caused by single genes, whereas it is abundantly clear that the genetic component of aging involves many different genes. Which ones would we select as targets for gene therapy? Obviously we would want to focus on genes whose actions could potentially affect the process of senescence itself in *all* cells—the housekeeping genes. First and foremost among these genes will likely be those involved in the generation and repair of oxidative cellular damage, such as the DNA helicase discussed earlier. We have already seen a form of this kind of gene therapy, involving the genes for the antioxidant enzymes superoxide dismutase and catalase, applied to fruit flies. By introducing extra copies of these genes, both average and maximal lifespans were significantly increased. Telomerase may eventually be a target for some limited forms of gene therapy, with the caveats already noted. We may also want to think of gene therapy using genes for natural proteins such as leptin, which suppress appetite, as an adjunct to some sort of caloric restriction regimen.

Will we want to go this far in our search for the fountain of youth? It is unlikely even to be proposed in the lifetime of anyone reading this book, but it is not at all beyond the realm of possibility. All of the elements of the technology for doing it are already in place. But in the meantime, there are other avenues to explore that could well have the same effect. As mentioned in the last section, we may not currently be experiencing the true maximal human lifespan for human beings because of excessive caloric intake. The general health benefits of a calorically restricted diet cannot be denied. Animals on calorically leaner diets have less disease, and by several measures age more slowly, than fully fed animals. The same results in larger animals could reasonably be expected.

But caloric restriction is only one approach. If we accept that aging of the organism is a reflection of the cumulative effects of cellular senescence, then the overall rate of decline after the breeding period will reflect a balance between the rates of cellular damage and cellular repair during that period. The evidence that this damage is to a great extent oxidative in nature has already been presented, and we have seen that the corresponding cellular repair mechanisms decline with age. We have also seen the evidence that caloric restriction reduces oxidative damage within the cell, and we also have good epidemiological and experimental evidence in hand that natural antioxidants taken in through diet can be effective in mitigating oxidative damage. The evidence that supplemental antioxidant vitamins taken alone are effective is less compelling at present, but that may be for lack of appropriately designed trials. Beyond doubt, cigarette smoke contains potent oxidants that can work their way into cells through the bloodstream and wreak oxidative damage; the overall health benefits of not smoking are by now self-evident, and could be a major factor in increasing human average lifespan worldwide.

The study of aging is one of the most exciting areas of contemporary biomedical research. More than any other human science, aging impinges on virtually every aspect of our biological existence, from our earliest beginnings as an embryo, through the intriguing interplay between senescence and reproduction in our middle years, and on into our never-ending battle to lessen the burden of growing old. The understanding of aging we have gained from the study of individuals and populations has been enormously advanced by our newfound ability to dissect aging at its most fundamental cellular and molecular levels. Like other technological advances, the new molecular approaches to human aging will generate problems as well as solutions. There are nay-sayers who would like to turn back the clock, or at least slow it down until we catch up with ourselves. But that is not, for better or worse, the way human beings go about their business. Molecular medicine will be an important part of our lives in the twenty-first century. Beyond doubt, it will enable us to continue learning more about how and why we age, and we will continue our efforts to increase both the quantity and the quality of human lifespan in the years ahead. This may require that we make adjustments in our thinking, and even in our social and political institutions. But we will do it. We will do it.

Bibliography

Chapter 1

Carey, J., et al. Slowing of mortality rates at older ages in large medfly cohorts. *Science* 258:457 (1992)

Hayflick, L. *How and Why We Age.* Ballantine Books, New York, 1994.

Hayflick, L. and P. Moorhead. The serial cultivation of human diploid cell strains. *Experimental Cell Research* 25:585 (1961).

Holiday, R. The current status of the protein error theory of aging. *Experimental Gerontology* 31:449 (1996)

McGue, M., et al. Longevity is moderately heritable in a sample of Danish twins born 1870–1880. *Journal of Gerontology* 48:B237 (1993)

Thoms, W. J. *Human Longevity.* Scriner, Welford and Armstrong, New York, 1873.

Weismann, August. *Essays Upon Heredity.* (E. Bottom, et al., eds) Oxford Press, 1891

Chapter 2

Bladier, C., et al. Response of a primary human fibroblast cell line to H_2O_2: senescence-like growth arrest or apoptosis? *Cell Growth and Differentiation* 8:589 (1997)

Chapter 3

Comfort, Alex. Biological aspects of senescence. *Biological Reviews* 29:284 (1954)

Comfort, Alex. *The Biology of Senescence.* Elsevier, New York. 3rd Edition, 1979

Cutler, R. Evolution of human longevity: a critical overview. *Mechanisms of Aging and Development* 9:337 (1979)

Finch, C. and M. Rose. Hormones and the physiological architecture of life history evolution. *The Quarterly Review of Biology* 70:1 (1995).

Fleming, J. and M. Rose. Genetics of Aging in Drosophila. *Handbook of the biology of aging.* Fourth ed. Academic Press, NY, 1996.

McEwen, B., et al. Ovarian steroids and the brain; implications for cognition and aging. *Neurology* 48:S8 (1997)

Murakami, S. and T. Johnson. A genetic pathway conferring life extension and resistance to UV stress in *Caenorhabditis elegans*. *Genetics* 143:1207 (1996)

Johnson, T. Genetic influences on aging. *Experimental Gerontology* 32:11 (1997)

Kirkwood, T. Repair and its evolution: survival vs. reproduction. In, *Physiological Ecology: An Evolutionary Approach to Resource Use.* Blackwell, London, 1981.

Kirkwood, T. and M. Rose. Evolution of senescence: late survival sacrificed for reproduction. *Philosophical Transactions of the Royal Society of London* B 332:15 (1991)

Partridge, L. and N. Barton. Optimality, mutation and the evolution of aging. *Nature* 362:305 (1993)

Reznick, D. Life history evolution in guppies (*Poecilia reticulata*) as a model for studying the evolutionary biology of aging. *Experimental Gerontology* 32:245 (1997)

Riggs, Jack E. Differential survival, natural selection and the manifestation of senescence. *Mechanisms of Aging and Development* 87:91 (1996).

Rose, Michael R. Laboratory evolution of postponed senescence in *Drosophila melanogaster*. *Evolution* 38:1004 (1984)

Williams, G. Pleiotropy, natural selection, and the evolution of senescence. *Evolution* 11:398 (1957)

Chapter 4

Brenner, S. The genetics of *Caenorhabditis elegans*. *Genetics* 77:71 (1974)

Driscoll, M. Cell death in *C. elegans*: molecular insights into mechanisms conserved between nematodes and mammals. *Brain Pathology* 6:411 (1996)

Ewbank, J., et al. Structural and functional conservation of the *Caenorhabditis elegans* timing gene clk-1. *Science* 275:980 (1997).

Friedman, D. and T. Johnson. A mutation in the *age-1* gene of *C. elegans* lengthens life and reduces hermaphrodite fertility. *Genetics* 118:75 (1988)

Klass, M. A method for the isolation of longevity mutants in the nematode *C. elegans* and initial results. *Mechanisms in Aging and Development* 22:279 (1983)

Lakowski, B. and S. Hekimi. Determination of lifespan in *Caenorhabditis elegans* by four clock genes. *Science* 272:1010 (1996)

Larsen, P. Aging and resistance to oxidative damage in *Caenorhabditis elegans*. *Proceedings of the National Academy of Science* 90:8905 (1993)

Lithgow, G. Molecular Genetics of *Caenorhabditis elegans* Aging. *Handbook of the Biology of Aging* (Fourth Edition). *Academic Press*, New York, 1996.

Chapter 5

Brown, W. Human mutations affecting aging. *Mechanisms of Aging and Development* 9:325 (1979)

Cockayne, E. Dwarfism with retinal atrophy and deafness. *Archives of Diseases in Childhood* 11:1 (1936)

DeBusk, F. The Hutchinson-Gilford progeria syndrome. *J. Pediatrics* 80:697 (1972)

Epstein, C., et al. Werner's syndrome: a review of its symptomology, natural history, pathological features, genetics and relationship to the natural aging process. *Medicine* 45:177 (1966)

Finch, C. and R. Tanzi. Genetics of Aging. *Science* 278:407 (1997)

Gray, M., et al. The Werner syndrome protein is a helicase. *Nature Genetics* 17:100 (1997).

Martin, G. Genetic syndromes in man with potential relevance to the pathobiology of aging. *Birth Defects* 14:5 (1978)

Martin, G. The genetics of aging. *Hospital Practice* February 15, 1997, p. 47.

Yu, C., et al. Positional cloning of the Werner's Syndrome gene. *Science* 272:258 (1996).

Chapter 6

Allsopp, R. Models of initiation of replicative senescence by loss of telomeric DNA. *Experimental Gerontology* 31:235 (1996)

Bodnar, A., et al. Extension of lifespan by introduction of telomerase into normal human cells. *Science* 279: 349–352 (1998)

Bond, J. et al. Evidence that transcriptional activation by p53 plays a direct role in the induction of cellular senescence. *Oncogene* 7:2097 (1996)

Brown, J., W. Wei and J. Sedivy. Bypass of senescence after disruption of p21CIP1/WAF1 gene in normal dipoid human fibroblasts. *Science* 277:831 (1997)

Campisi, J., et al. Control of replicative senescence. *Handbook of the Biology of Aging.* Academic Press, Inc., New York, 1996

Chiu, C. and C. Harley. Replicative senescence and cell immortality: the role of telomeres and telomerase. *Proceedings of the Society for Experimental Biology and Medicine* 214:99 (1997.)

Daniel, C. Aging of cells during serial propagation in vivo. *Advanced Gerontological Research* 4:167 (1972).

Gilley, D. and E. Blackburn. Lack of telomere shortening during senescence in Paramecium. *Proceedings of the National Academy of Sciences* 91:1955 (1994)

Goldstein, S. Replicative senescence: the human fibroblast comes of age. *Science* 249:1129 (1990)

Heichman, K. and J. Roberts. Rules to replicate by. *Cell* 79:557 (1994).

Ikram, Z., et al. The biological clock that measures the mitotic lifespan of mouse embryo fibroblasts continues to function in the presence of SV40 large tumor antigen. *Proceedings of the National Academy of Sciences* 91:6448 (1994)

Kastan, M., et al. Participation of p53 protein in the cellular response to DNA damage. *Cancer Research* 51:6304 (1991)

Kruk, P., et al. DNA damage and repair in telomeres: relation to aging. *Proceedings of the National Academy of Sciences* 92:258 (1995)

Magzars, G. and P. Jat. Expression of p24, a novel p21-related protein, correlates with measurement of the finite proliferative potential of rodent embryo fibroblasts. *Proceedings of the National Academy of Sciences* 94:151 (1997)

Olovnikov, A. Telomeres, telomerase and aging: origin of the theory. *Experimental Gerontology* 31:443 (1996)

Vaziri, H. and S. Benchimol. From telomere loss to p53 induction and activation of a DNA damage pathway at senescence. *Experimental Gerontology* 31:295

Weinberg, R. A. The retinoblastoma protein and cell cycle control. *Cell* 81:323 (1995).

West, M., et al. Replicative senescence of human skin fibroblasts correlates with a loss of regulation of collagenase activity. *Experimental Cell Research* 184:138 (1989)

Wright, W., et al. Telomerase activity in human germline and embryonic tissues and cells. *Developmental Genetics* 18:173 (1996)

Chapter 7

Donehower, L., et al. Mice deficient for p53 are developmentally normal but susceptible to spontaneous tumors. *Nature* 356:215 (1992).

Savatier, P. et al. Contrasting patterns of retinoblastoma protein expression in mouse embryonic stem cells and embryonic fibroblasts. *Oncogene* 9: 809 (1994))

Serrano, M., et al. Oncogenic ras provokes premature cell senescence associated with accumulation of p53 and p16. *Cell* 88:593 (1997)

Chapter 8

Cefalu, W., et al. A study of caloric restriction and cardiovascular aging in cynomolgus monkeys: a potential model for aging research. *Journals of Gerontology* (Biological Science) 52A:B10 (1997)

Dunn, S., et al. Dietary restriction reduces insulin-like growth factor-1 levels, which modulates apoptosis, cell proliferation and tumor progression in p53-deficient mice. *Cancer Research* 57:4667 (1997)

Hass, B. et al. Dietary restriction in humans: report on the Little Rock Conference on the value, feasibility and parameters of a proposed study. *Mechanisms of Aging and Development* 91:79 (1996)

Masoro, E. and S. Austad. The evolution of the antiaging action of dietary restriction: A hypothesis. *Journals of Gerontology* 51A:B387 (1996)

McCay, C., M. Crowell and L. Maynard. The effect of retarded growth upon the length of lifespan and upon the ultimate body size. *Journal of Nutrition* 10:63 (1935)

Miller, R. A. The aging immune system: primer and prospectus. *Science* 273:70 (1996)

Pendergrass, W., et al. Caloric restriction: conservation of cellular replicative capacity in vitro accompanies lifespan extension in mice. *Experimental Cell Research* 217:309 (1995).

Ramsey, J., et al. Energy expenditure of adult male rhesus monkeys during the first 30 months of dietary restriction. *American Journal of Physiology* 272:E901 (1997)

Spaulding, C., et al. The accumulation of non-replicative, non-functional senescent T cells with age is avoided in calorically restricted mice by an enhancement of T cell apoptosis. *Mechanisms of Aging and Development* 93:25 (1997)

Velthuis-te Wierik, E., et al. Energy restriction: a useful intervention to retard human aging? Results of a feasability study. *European Journal of Clinical Nutrition* 48:138 (1994)

Walford, R. *Maximum Life Span.* W. W. Norton, New York, 1983.

Weindruch, R. and R. Walford. *The Retardation of Aging and Disease by Dietary Restriction.* Charles C. Thomas, Springfield, 1988.

Chapter 9

Ames, B., et al. Oxidants, antioxidants and the degenerative diseases of aging. *Proceedings of the National Academy of Sciences* 90:7915 (1993)

Balasz, L., and M. Leon. Evidence of an oxidative challenge in the Alzheimer's brain. *Neurochemical Research* 19:1131 (1994).

Block, G., et al. Fruit, vegetables and cancer prevention: a review of the epidemiological evidence. *Nutrition and Cancer* 18:1 (1992)

Buring, J. and C. Hennekens. Antioxidant vitamins and cardiovascular disease. *Nutrition Reviews* 55 (Supplement):S53 (1997)

Chen, Q. and B. Ames. Senescence-like growth arrest induced by hydrogen peroxide in human diploid fibroblast F65 cells. *Proceedings of the National Academy of Sciences* 91:4130 (1994)

Chen, Q., et al. Oxidative DNA damage and senescence of human diploid fibroblasts. *Proceedings of the National Academy of Sciences* 92:4337 (1995).

Feuers, R., et al. Caloric restriction, aging, and antioxidant enzymes. *Mutation Research* 295:191 (1993)

Haley-Zitlin, V. and A. Richardson. Effect of dietary restriction on DNA repair and DNA damage. *Mutation Research* 237:245 (1993)

Halliwell, B. Antioxidants and human disease: a general introduction. *Nutrition Reviews* 55 (Supplement II):S44 (1997)

Kimmick, G., et al. Vitamin E and breast cancer: a review. *Nutrition and Cancer* 27:109 (1997)

Kruk, P., et al. DNA damage and repair in telomeres: relation to aging. *Proceedings of the National Academy of Sciences* 92:258 (1995)

Kushi, L., et al. Dietary antioxidant vitamins and death from coronary heart disease in post-menopausal women. *New England Journal of Medicine* 334:1156 (1996)

Lane, M. et al. Calorie restriction lowers body temperature in rhesus monkeys, consistent with a postulated anti-aging mechanisms in rodents. *Proceedings of the National Academy of Sciences* 93:4159 (1996)

Larsen, P. Aging and resistance to oxidative damage in *Caenorhabditis elegans*. *Proceedings of the National Academy of Science* 90:8905 (1992)

Lindahl, T., et al. DNA excision repair pathways. *Current Opinion in Genetics and Development* 7:158 (1997)

Miquel, J. An update on the oxygen stress-mitochondrial mutation theory of aging: genetic and evolutionary implications. *Experimental Gerontology* 33:113 (1998)

Omenn, G., et al. Effects of a combination of beta-carotene and vitamin A on lung cancer and cardiovascular disease. *New England Journal of Medicine* 334:1150 (1996)

Orr, W. and R. Sohal. Extension of life-span by overexpression of superoxide dismutase and catalase in *Drosophila melanogaster*. *Science* 263:1128 (1994)

Rimm, E., et al. Vitamin E consumption and the risk of coronary heart disease in men. *New England Journal of Medicine* 328:1450 (1993)

Shikenaga, M., et al. Oxidative damage and mitochondrial decay in aging. *Proceedings of the National Academy of Sciences* 91:10771 (1994)

Sohal, R. and R. Weindruch. Oxidative stress, caloric restriction, and aging. *Science* 273:59 (1996).

Stampfer, M. et al. Vitamin E consumption and the risk of coronary disease in women. *New England Journal of Medicine* 328:1444 (1993)

Szilard, L. On the nature of the aging process. *Proceedings of the National Academy of Sciences* 45:30 (1959).

Tolmasoff, J., T. Ono and R. Cutler. Superoxide dismutase: correlation with lifespan and specific metabolic rate in primate species. *Proceedings of the National Academy of Science* 77:2777 (1980)

von Zglinicki, T., et al. Mild hyperoxia shortens telomeres and inhibits proliferation of fibroblasts: A model for senescence? *Experimental Cell Research* 220:186 (1995)

Walford, R., et al. The calorically restricted low-fat nutrient-dense diet in Biosphere 2 significantly lowers blood glucose, total leukocyte count, cholesterol and blood pressure in humans. *Proceedings of the National Academy of Sciences* 89:11533 (1992)

Wei, Q., et al. DNA repair and aging in basal cell carcinoma: a molecular epidemiology study. *Proc. Nat'l. Acad. Sci.* 90:1614 (1993).

Weirich-Schweiger, H., et al. Correlation between senescence and DNA repair in cells from young and old individuals, and in premature aging syndromes. *Mutation Research* 316:37 (1994)

Weraarchakul, N., et al. The effect of aging and dietary restriction on DNA repair. *Experimental Cell Research* 181:197 (1989)

Yuan, H., et al. Increased susceptibility of late passage human diploid fibroblasts to oxidative stress. *Experimental Gerontology* 31:465 (1996)

Chapter 10

Berezovska, O., et al. Developmental regulation of presenilin mRNA expression parallels notch expression. *Journal of Neuropathology and Experimental Neurology* 56:40 (1997).

Butterfield, D., et al. Free radical oxidation of brain proteins in acclerated senescence and its modulation by *N*-tert-butyl-a-phenylnitrone. *Proceedings of the National Academy of Sciences* 94:674 (1997)

Carney, J., et al. Reversal of age-related increase in brain protein oxidation, decrease in enzyme activity, and loss of temporal and spatial memory by chronic administration of the spin-trapping compound *N*-tert-butyl-a-phenylnirone. *Proceedings of the National Academy of Science* 88:3633 (1991)

Dubey, A., et al. Effect of age and caloric intake on protein oxidation in different brain regions and on behavioral functions of the mouse. *Archives of Biochemistry and Biophysics* 333:189 (1996)

Edelberg, H. and J. Wei. The biology of Alzheimer's disease. *Mechanisms of Aging and Development* 91:95 (1996)

Hardy, John. Amyloid, the presenilins and Alzheimer's disease. *Trends in Neuroscience* 20:154 (1997)

Hensley, K., et al. Reactive oxygen species as causal agents in the neurotoxicity of the Alzheimer's disease-associated amyloid beta-peptide. *Annals of the New York Academy of Science* 786:120 (1996)

Jarvik, L., et al. Organic brain syndrome and aging: a six-year followup of twins. *Archives of General Psychiatry* 37:280 (1980)

Jeong, S., et al. Age-related changes in expression of Alzheimer's ß-APP in the brain of senescence-accelerated mouse SAM-10. *Neuroreport* 8:1733 (1997).

Katzman, R. and T. Saitoh. Advances in Alzheimer's disease. *FASEB Journal* 5:278

Morrison, J. and P. Hof. Life and death of neurons in the aging brain. *Science* 278:412 (1997)

Levitan, D., et al. Assessment of normal and mutant human presenilin function in *Caenorhabditis elegans*. *Proceedings of the National Academy of Sciences* 93:14940 (1996)

Miyamoto, M. Characteristics of age-related behavioral changes in senescence-accelerated mouse SAMP8 and SAMP9. *Experimental Gerontology* 32:139 (1997)

Morris, C., et al. Molecular biology of APO E alleles in Alzheimer's and non-

Alzheimer's dementias. *Journal of Neurological Transmission* (Suppl) 47:205 (1996)

Takeda, T., et al. Senescence-accelerated mouse (SAM): a novel murine model of accelerated senescence. *Journal of the American Geriatric Society* 39:911 (1991)

Wong, P., et al. Presenilin 1 is required for notch-1 and D11-1 expression in the paraxial mesoderm. *Nature* 387:288 (1997)

Chapter 11

Austad, S. *Why We Age.* John Wiley and Sons, New York, 1997.

Gray, M. The Werner syndrome protein is a DNA helicase. *Nature Genetics* 17:100 (1997)

Sinclair, D., K. Mills and L. Guarente. Accelerated aging and nucleolar fragmentation in yeast *Sgs1* mutants. *Science* 277:1313 (1997)

Kannisto, V. Development of oldest-old mortality, 1950–1990: Evidence from 28 developed countries. *Monographs on Population Aging.* Odense University Press, 1994.

Index

A NOTE ON THE TYPE

A Means to an End is set in Adobe Caslon, a font drawn by Carol Twombly in 1989. Twombly's digitized version is based on the work of English engraver William Caslon, who was active in the early eighteenth century. More old style than modern, Caslon's work is an extension of Nicolas Jenson's fifteenth-century type cutting; his font has since been considered the work of a master and has been one of the most popular and widely used typefaces in the history of the printed word.

Composition by David Thorne.